"I can't give you a higher recommendation than to put your [...] Sanderson and learn from her. She understands exactly what [...] you are now to where you want to be."

- **John Assaraf, 'New York Times' best-selling author of 'Innercise', 'Having It All' and 'The Answer', and world-leading mindset and behaviour expert**

'It has been a pleasure working with you on your "Online Brand Assessment". It gave me a deeper appreciation and understanding of your thoughts, process, goals and challenges. I was very impressed with your background, business ideas, intelligence, experience, and friendly personality.'

- **Howard Lim, Fortune 500, President of How Creative**

'Mutu sponsored many of Caroline's events and saw first-hand how much her mindfulness training was really welcomed by attendees, we saw so many business owners sign up to Caroline's training. Caroline has a unique way of inspiring the audience and catching their imagination with her mindful training, at the end of the course it left them feeling like they could take on the world. I wouldn't hesitate to recommend Caroline and her team no matter what type of business you're involved with.'

- **Barry Stephens, Managing Director, Mutu Ltd, Chairman Fellowship of British Hairdressing**

'Caroline Sanderson is hugely inspirational and a joy to work with – we have watched her develop over the last few years and were thrilled when she joined our roster for PR at the start of 2020. She is a visionary with some of the most incredible ideas, she is driven and has enjoyed well-deserved success as a result. Straight talking and results motivated – every salon needs Caroline in their life to help them take control and propel their own business forward.'

- **Sally Learmouth, Director, Gloss Communications**

'Good Salon Guide was proud to award Salon Jedi Academy with a 5 Star Good Training Guide, the first ever for a digital training platform and it's a fantastic platform for business owners to take advantage of Caroline's hard-won, and proven, business and marketing advice.'

- **Gareth Penn, Director, GSG**

'Caroline Sanderson to me is a genuine person with excellent advice based on her experience and knowledge. She is inspirational as a businesswoman that has had the same problems as me and come out the other side smiling. Her ideas are amazing and best of all.....they work! The support network that Caroline has created is something I don't think I could be without now. After 5 months as a Profit Partner, compared to the previous year results are phenomenal.

Retail Growth
- November **up 87%**
- December **up 40%**
- January **up 66%**
- February **up 6%** (I was off salon floor with broken wrist)
- March **up 27%**

Service Growth
- December **up 12%**
- January **up 7%**
- February **up 5%**
- March **up 10%**

There has been a huge change in our private lives too, going from rented accommodation with no savings to buying our first home , just having a 4-bed detached built now which will be ready for January..... exactly one year since we decided to follow Salon Jedi Profit Partners training to see if we could get our dream home......and we have done it! Thanks Caroline.'

- ***Emma Simmons, Salon 54***

'A quick update on my sales from last week. Total £2,080 from one email. This week I will use packages again to get more business through Facebook. I know that I will get another £1,270 on packages. 90% of clients went for the highest-priced option, there was a lower-priced option. Prices were £40 to £60 more than usual, so I am making double on every cut and blow dry by calling them Ultimate Redesign for the cost of shampoo & conditioner.

£2,080 is more than we would take in any one week, other than Christmas. Really chuffed and really excited about further and future possibilities. As I think I said I woke up last Tuesday morning going bust, but by Wednesday morning the month's bills had been covered. Thank you (and Salon Jedi Training)! xx'

- ***Jenny Curry, Sensational Hair***

'I attended a Salon Jedi bootcamp on March 10th, I remember as it was my birthday. I had seen the Facebook advert and listened to Caroline's story which resonated with my own. I remember thinking what a remarkable woman, what's her secret?

I loved every minute of it. She was super focused and grabbed the audience as they waited in anticipation of what was coming next. For the first time in many years I felt I had hope. I knew in the first hour I was hungry for more and eagerly signed up for the two-day training school. Along I went with a brand new laptop under my arm and a terrified yet exciting feeling as I knew computers were not my best friend. We covered mindset and business marketing, wow it was amazing.

That day I decided to take action and signed up for the full package. This would enable me to get a new more modern website, access to group chats, mastermind calls, one-to-one coaching calls, online business school and Caroline and Carla would come to my salon.

I left there that day equipped with the tools to finally turn my almost 16-year-old business into a profit-making salon. The day came when Caroline and Carla walked through my salon doors and turned the place upside down then the right way up again. Caroline worked with me and Carla worked with the staff. In two days they had made such a shift it was noticeable with the clients and the whole team became motivated.

Two days after they left the salon, we saw a 261% increase in sales because we implemented the changes they had put in place. Then sales increased the next month by £1,000, then £2,000 the month after that and kept growing.

In December 2019 we banked 400% more than any other year. 2019 saw the biggest turnover in 16 years of trading. Caroline and her amazing team gave me the confidence to get my teaching certificate and open my second business.

All I can say is I know I'm in a much better place today than I know I would have been. I can sleep at night now someone has my back. I will be forever grateful. Thank you Caroline and Salon Jedi. Xxx'

- **Amanda Allan, Heavenly Sensations**

'I have made an EXTRA £10,963.50 since joining Salon Jedi 14 weeks ago. Not bad, eh? To say I'm on my own plus one new stylist I had to take on since starting Salon Jedi? I'm really pleased, and I also just bought myself a new car and paid cash for it which is fantastic.'

- **Clare Pearson, Ash Hair**

'That moment when you glimpse what you have always dreamed about, happened after the first part of education from Salon Jedi Lite.

I have been in hairdressing for 34 years and dreamed of a salon that loved people, loved hair and made money. I have written in many dreambooks, set targets and goals but seemed to have always struggled to push past certain points. I have been on courses and all sorts to discover the "secret" or "reason", but to no avail. Please don't misunderstand, I have had a successful business for most of those years in terms of profit, which by most accounts is a great thing! But I have always dreamed of a salon that had five star customer service, a team that worked together and towards becoming better and better in hairdressing skills and personal development, and a business that ran with systems and procedures.

We have found all this in the education that comes from Caroline and the Salon Jedi team. They have helped us discover who we are, what we are about, where we are going and helped us to dream again in our business.

As an example, Caroline teaches many strategies to help you build your business, but the first one we tried was a Conditioning Treatment bundle and we followed the Salon Jedi way to the letter (as much as I could, we had only just begun!) and in one email we sold 28 packages @£67 each, making £1,876. **THIS WAS MY LIGHT-BULB MOMENT!** *Bearing in mind, in a year we had sold two conditioning treatments, this was ZERO to 28 in one email.*

The vouchers are all part of our strategy learned from Salon Jedi and will lead to further sales if all are taken up:
28 Kerastraight treatments = £3,500
28 Half price intense boosts = £378
Lots and lots of experience for our apprentices = PRICELESS

from ZERO TO £5,754 in one email – not too shabby!

Alongside the mindset education, the missing piece in my experience, you realise that you can do this, achieve the dream you've always wanted, know what you want and how to achieve it! Dream Again!'

- **Darren Mitzi, Darren Michael Hairdressing**

'Caroline and her team have bagged over 100 award nominations and wins and 2020 sees the launch of her M.I.N.D.F.U.L. Salon Source Code, teaching salons a 4-part solution covering mindset, marketing, management and maintenance to grow their business and put systems in place to ensure ongoing success without salon owners having to be on the salon floor to oversee everything.'

- **Salonnv.co.uk**

'I have worked for and with Caroline for eight years and it has been the most amazing journey and life-changing experience. Not only is she my employer but I regard her as an inspirational mentor and friend. I know without her guidance and support I would not have been able to achieve my goals or even believe I could have such goals to reach. I can honestly say that Caroline has made the most positive impact in my life and her generosity and guidance and belief in me means I cannot fail, and I am excited and focused to carry on working with her for years to come.'

- **Carla Zebrowski, Salon Managing Director & Salon Jedi Coach**

'I have had great inspiration and learning by working with Caroline for the past nine years. By focusing on growth mindset, it has helped me become one of the busiest stylists within the salon which I am extremely grateful for. She knows how to bring the best out of her team by inspiring and mentoring them.'

- **Louise Cameron, Ego Hair Design**

'After joining Salon Jedi Academy in April 2020, I learnt about a different style of Facebook advert through the academy courses and Caroline's coaching. I decided to create a Facebook Messenger Engagement Advert post the COVID-19 lockdown, which led to fabulous success. The aim was to create an interest database and, as a result, a better process for our Front of House team. This gave the Front of House team a pre-populated client interest list in an Excel database, who they could contact to arrange appointments. It helped the reception process go extremely smoothly and improved standards. I've seen the following results:

Cost of Advert: *£9.37*
Type of Advert: *Branded Facebook Messenger Engagement Advert*
Date of Advert: *Started at end of June 2020*
Advert subject and goal: *Promoting reopening after Lockdown to people who had engaged via Messenger over the past year and link to a Google Form designed as a Waiting List Booking Request form*
Impressions: *737*
Responses: *208*
Value of Advert Responses: *£13,014.13 (£4k of which was vouchers redeemed)'*

- **Lisa McCrink, Zen Day Spa**

'I personally am a big believer in the idea that you can hold yourself back by your own narrative. Caroline explores this concept extensively with some great ideas on how you can challenge and change that.'

- **Jack Howard, Award-Winning Global Colour Educator & Podcaster**

'After reading just one chapter I've gone straight into the salon and made some tweaks - this book has really helped me to refocus and reinforced the benefits of a positive mindset.'

- **Karine Jackson, London Hairdresser of Year 2007/President of the Fellowship for British Hairdressing 2017-2019**

"Caroline's perspective on the importance of mindset and her achievable tips for financial success make this book a must for any salon owner."

- **Errol Douglas MBE**

ISBN: 9798679560703
Imprint: Independently published
©2020 Caroline Sanderson. Salon Jedi Limited.

This work was produced in collaboration with Write Business Results Limited. For more information on Write Business Results' business book, blog and podcast services, please visit www.writebusinessresults.com or email your query to info@writebusinessresults.com.

Dream BIG !

Love Caroline x

THE SALON JEDI

The Big Business Breakthrough For Ambitious Salon Owners

by Caroline Sanderson

ACKNOWLEDGEMENTS

Thank you's:

Andy Harrington for writing the foreword.

Team Ego past and present who have all played a part in my journey.

Team Jedi who helped make the book possible, and to all our Salon Jedis and associates who gave the case studies and testimonials.

To all my mentors who inspire me to follow my mission to educate and empower ambitious salon owners to become leaders and masters of their own mind and business for more profits and more freedom.

DEDICATION

This book is dedicated to my three beautiful children, Lois, Buster and Dixie, who inspire me daily. I love you.

And to my rock-star family, I couldn't do what I do or have written this book without your support.

And for every salon owner out there feeling stuck, stagnant or downright stressed out, let this book be the light at the end of your tunnel.

Caroline x

CONTENTS

FOREWORD

I first met Caroline in July 2018, when she joined my Professional Speakers Academy as a student. While she completed her training, I also coached Caroline on a one-to-one basis and it was during these sessions that we got to know each other.

The thing that struck me most was her drive to act on what she was learning. She understood that knowledge is nothing without implementation. You can learn all the knowledge in the world, but if you don't implement it you aren't going to see the results you want. Caroline has an incredible ability to take what she learns and turn that into action, which very quickly delivers exceptional results.

Of all the students I've had over the years, there is only a small percentage who have had the same level of results that Caroline has had in such a short space of time. These results speak for themselves.

I put this down to her mindset. Mindset is so important in business, and I know it's a topic that Caroline will talk about throughout this book.

If you're wondering what you can learn from Caroline and her success, it's mindset and implementation. I always recommend that if you see someone who is getting the results that you want, you should model them. This book will introduce you to the model of what Caroline does so well and I suggest that you read it, take note and use this to model her and get the results that you want.

Success is, of course, subjective and can mean different things to different people. If success for you means creating a highly profitable salon business that doesn't rely on you, and expanding into other areas to give you multiple streams of income, then Caroline is the picture of success.

If that's the kind of success you are looking for, she is an excellent person to listen to and learn from. She has been there and done it, and now she's sharing her knowledge and the steps it takes to get there in this book. With this as a resource, you can model those steps and start seeing results in your salon too.

Andy Harrington
Sunday Times Best-Selling Author
Passion Into Profit

INTRODUCTION

Welcome to the beginning of your journey towards creating the sustainable, profitable and high-performing salon you've always wanted. I know from my own experience how rewarding but also how tough it can be at times to own and manage a salon. Within the hair and beauty industry, it's all too common for salon owners to work all the hours God sends, but feel as though they have very little to show for it. If you've picked up this book because you're looking for some help to not only make your salon more profitable but to also give yourself more freedom, you're in the right place.

My name is Caroline Sanderson. I'm the owner of Ego Hair Design in Inverness and I established the Salon Jedi Academy to help empower ambitious salon owners like you to master your salon business for more profits, more time and more freedom. In the following chapters, I'll be sharing the knowledge I've gained from setting up my own salon and going from working a full column and managing it, to having a highly profitable business that runs without me needing to set foot on the salon floor.

I'll talk you through the four key principles you will need to master to find your own freedom and build the salon and the culture that you want for your business. These four principles are mindset, marketing, management and maintenance. The parts of this book aren't exhaustive, but they are designed to get you started on your journey towards having an even more successful salon.

When you finish reading this book I want you to feel empowered to take the next steps. Believe me, I understand what it feels like when you don't think you have control of your salon, and what it's like to feel completely trapped. I'll share more of my personal story as we go through the book. What I want you to know right now is that you don't have to feel like this forever. Having a successful salon and leading a better, more balanced life is within your control.

Working on yourself is an essential first step, and it's why this book begins by talking about mindset. When you commit to working on yourself daily and create an empowering mindset, you'll find other elements begin to fall into place. Once you have created the foundations with your mindset, I'll delve into the marketing, management and maintenance elements of building, maintaining and eventually scaling or selling a successful, thriving, happy salon.

This book is offering you a starting point to upgrade your mindset and upgrade your skill set. It's important to work on both of these to progress, but once you do you'll find that results quickly follow.

Your marketing skills are essential because it's these that will help you bring customers through your doors. This isn't only about attracting new customers, but also about bringing back your existing customers time and time again.

If you already own a salon, you have probably realised that you can't do everything and this is where management comes in. As your salon starts to get busier and busier, you need to make sure it's being managed properly, either by you or by someone else.

Finally, I'll talk about maintenance, because a salon won't keep performing at a high level and stay highly profitable without some work to keep it there. What I'm going to help you realise is that this doesn't require a lot of your time, provided you create the right culture and put the right systems in place.

By the end of this book, you'll have a framework that you can use to start making positive changes to your life and your salon. You'll know where you can go for help and guidance to take your salon to the next level. Although I refer to hair salons throughout the book, because this is what I own, this information is transferable to any salon or small business.

An essential first step is taking responsibility for the situation you are in right now. I know it can be difficult to look around and accept that you are the creator of everything you're seeing and experiencing right now, especially if your business is struggling. However, it's important to understand that what you see in your salon is a reflection of what you put out into the world. The good thing is that you have the power to change this. Everything you see comes from you! That means with a bit of guidance and the right attitude, you can build your salon into the business you've always wanted it to be. Let's get started.

PART 1

MINDSET

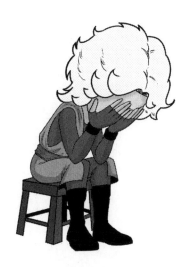

I've worked with hundreds of salon owners in my career and I can always tell exactly what an owner's mindset is going to be like just from looking at their results. I won't necessarily have met them in person, I won't have been to their salon, but I can tell you what kind of mindset they'll have. You might be wondering how, and it's really not rocket science, but I can tell you that your mindset will be reflected in the results that you're achieving.

I'm also going to tell you right now that your mindset is the most important factor in your success as a salon owner. Mindset comes above your training, your skills as a hairdresser, where you have your salon and who you have working for you. This is why I'm introducing you to mindset right at the beginning of this book, because it really is that important.

In the following chapters, I'll explain the two types of mindset I generally encounter – fixed mindsets and growth mindsets – and also how you can tell which of these mindsets you have (or are currently closer to). It's really important to understand that there's no judgement, blame or shame around your mindset. It is so deeply rooted in your subconscious you are probably not even aware of it yourself. What I want to do in these chapters is help you assess your own mindset and understand how changing it could be hugely beneficial for your business.

Once you've identified your mindset, I'll give you some advice and tools to help you change it. That's the wonderful thing about your mindset; it can be changed. Even if you realise that you have a fixed mindset that is currently holding you back, don't worry. As soon as you identify it, you're one step closer to making positive changes that will make you happier and help your business thrive.

By the time you finish reading this part of the book I want you to feel empowered to make a change. I want you to believe in yourself and your ability to change your mindset for the better. Is that going to be easy? No! Is it going to be worthwhile? Absolutely. To change your business you have to start by changing yourself. This book will help you upgrade your mindset and upgrade your skills; but your mindset is the foundation of your business, which is why we're starting here.

CHAPTER 1

FIXED MINDSET VS GROWTH MINDSET

I'd like to begin by sharing the stories of two female salon owners. Imagine that they both have their salons on the same street in the same town and that they both have the same years of experience and opened their salons at the same time. As you'll quickly realise, the difference is mindset.

MEET SANDRA...

As Sandra walks into her salon in the morning, she sighs. It's empty again with no customers and her team are standing around talking. She says a brief 'good morning' to her team before going into the back office. *How am I going to pay their wages when we don't have any customers? I can't keep this up. I'm not making any money. I wasn't cut out for this.* As thoughts start running through her head, Sandra feels the panic rising inside and a sick feeling settles in her stomach. *This is all my fault. I'm not doing enough to bring in new customers. But how can I get more new customers when I'm not good at marketing? Every time I try it never works! No one is spending money on haircuts and treatments at the moment. What am I going to do? I just want to give up.*

This is Sandra's inner story all morning. It's running through her head while she's working in the office, trying to balance the figures. Feeling completely disillusioned, she comes back onto the floor. It's a little after 12pm and the salon is about to hit its busy lunchtime spell. She notices a customer waiting by the desk, and then realises that one of her stylists hasn't turned up. She was supposed to be working at 12pm. *Staff have been calling in sick a lot lately...* Sandra doesn't let this thought finish. She calls the stylist but only reaches her voicemail. She checks the diary and realises she'll need to cover the column that day for a few hours. *Not ideal when it's meant to be my day in the office, but I need the customers. I can't just turn them away because my stylist is sick.*

At around 2pm, the missing stylist waltzes in. She offers a vague explanation as to why she was late. Sandra is just relieved she's shown up at all and takes the opportunity to retreat to the office. She knows she should talk to her stylist about showing up on time and give her a final warning for her lateness, it's not the first time. I can't face a confrontation today. I'll deal with it another time. *I can't afford to lose a stylist right now, better to have someone than no one at all for that chair.*

Sandra struggles to concentrate on her work for the rest of the day. She was going to update her salon's social media pages but she doesn't have the energy. Her negative self-talk keeps resurfacing and pulling her focus away from the business. She feels drained and completely out of her depth. *We're not getting enough clients through the door. This is just a small town. I can't find more clients.* She leaves the office as her team are finishing up for the day. Before she leaves and locks up, she checks the next day's diary. Her heart sinks even more when she sees all the white space. The only clients booked in the next morning are in her own column. As she leaves she gives her team a half smile. *I hope we have some clients tomorrow morning...*

MEET JENNY...

When Jenny arrives at her salon in the morning there are no customers. Her team are standing around talking and Jenny greets them with a beaming smile. She goes into the office and checks the diary. No clients are booked in until 11am. *How can we get the salon to fill up a bit earlier?* She starts to wonder if there is anything she can do to encourage clients to book earlier appointments, or to attract clients who would like those early slots. She takes out her laptop and starts doing some research on targeted social media advertising. *I wonder if there's something I'm missing? Something I'm not doing?* Just then, one of her stylists pops her head around the door and asks if Jenny can train her on how to use the new booking system before they get busy. Jenny smiles, 'Sure!'

At 11.50am, Jenny realises one of her stylists hasn't arrived yet. She is due to start work at 12pm. Jenny pops back to the office and calls her, only reaching her voicemail. She leaves her a message telling her to contact her as soon as she can. *She's been calling in sick a lot lately. I can't keep covering and rearranging her appointments. I'll need to talk to her.*

A quick glance at the diary shows that they'll be stretched for the next few hours. With a bit of clever rearranging, she manages to get all the clients moved to her other stylists so she can carry on working in the office and focus on developing the new morning booking strategy. Although it takes some time out of her day, she's pleased that she doesn't have to cover a column. *I've still got a good couple of hours this afternoon to work on my marketing plan.*

The missing stylist turns up two hours late. Jenny hears her arrive, takes a deep breath and takes her into the back office to have a chat. *These conversations are never easy, but it's not fair on me or the rest of the team if she's going to keep behaving like this.* Jenny has a conversation with her about being on time and explains that she's letting her and the rest of the team down, and the effect it has on the rest of the team and clients. She asks her yet again if there is anything wrong and whether she really wants to work there and gets an evasive answer. She gives her a final warning for her lateness; it's the third time in a month. *She'll probably quit before I let her go, but better that than having someone unreliable on the team. I would rather have less of the right staff than more of the wrong staff.*

Although it quietens down in the afternoon, Jenny feels as though she's accomplished a lot. She has set up some new targeted local adverts on social media and has updated her marketing plan. *One day that salon floor will be bustling from 9am to 6pm.* She smiles to herself as she pictures the scene and imagines not being able to hear the radio over the noise of hairdryers and chatter between her stylists and customers. She spends the final hour of her day looking up and contacting potential business mentors. *I know I can make this salon a huge success, I just need a little extra help to get there.*

As Jenny leaves for the day, she thanks her team for their support and for stepping in to manage the extra work due to the late and missing stylist. She also reminds the team of the training session she's arranged for the next morning because there are no clients in. Although she's tired, she's excited. Reaching out to potential mentors was a little scary, but she knows it will make all the difference to the future of the business. *I can't wait to see if anyone has replied tomorrow!* She's still thinking of a busy and bustling salon as she walks down the street.

These two examples might be slightly simplified, but they're designed to show you what a difference a growth mindset makes compared to a fixed mindset. In the rest of this chapter I'll unpack the characteristics of each mindset for you, but refer back to these stories as well. I'm sure you can see which of these two women has the fixed mindset and which has the growth mindset.

In the first example we meet Sandra, who has a fixed mindset. She is stressed. She's not happy. She feels overwhelmed and she lacks direction for her business. This isn't how you want to or should feel after a day at work. Without changing her mindset, she will stay in the same position, facing the same problems, or will simply give up on her business.

In the second example we meet Jenny, who has a growth mindset. She knows she has some issues, but she's in control. She's looking for solutions. She feels excited for the future, because she knows what she wants it to look like. She's determined to do what it takes to realise her vision of a busy and thriving salon. Leaving your salon with a smile on your face, even after a challenging day, is what you want.

Notice the difference between the inner dialogues of each woman. We are only ever doing two things with our inner dialogue: asking questions or making statements. Sandra asked disempowering questions like, 'How can I get more clients when I'm no good?' and made statements like, 'We're not getting enough clients.' Compare that to Jenny, who asked, 'Where can I find a mentor to help me?' and made statements like, 'I know I can make this salon a huge success.'

WHERE DOES YOUR MINDSET COME FROM?

Your mindset is something that's rooted deeply in your subconscious. It's not something you just wake up with one day, it's created gradually over the days, weeks, months and years of your life. A lot of it is controlled by your subconscious limiting beliefs, which we are often completely unaware of until we start to focus our attention on our mindset.

Our awareness of 'self' starts at around two years old, and by the time you are around seven years old, your self-identity is formed. We carry many subconscious beliefs about ourselves, and many of these were put in place when we were a very young child and affect us to this day.

These limiting beliefs cause us to turn our focus inwards. We blame others and shame ourselves (self-blame) when things don't go to plan. I'll talk more about limiting beliefs and how you can deal with them in the next chapter.

Another major factor in your mindset is fear. The trouble with fear is that it leads you to make bad decisions, or it means you avoid making decisions at all. The brain has no clarity in a fear state. It is ready for fight or flight only and loses the ability for creative, solutions-focused thought.

For example, you might be scared of confrontation, which in turn means you are scared of dealing with difficult team members, taking control of your salon and leading your team. If you have this fear of confrontation, then you'll make decisions that involve you avoiding confrontation (flight), or you may get angry and deal with the situation in the wrong way (fight). This often isn't good for you or your business. If there are issues in your staffroom but you're scared of confrontation, you will more than likely avoid them. The longer you leave it, the more out of control you feel, which makes you feel more fearful and the cycle continues.

When you feel like this, it won't matter how hard you're working, because you will always feel like you're not getting anywhere. Just as you feel as though you're making progress, something else will seem to happen to bring you back down. It can feel like Groundhog Day.

What I want to help you realise in this chapter, and the chapters that follow, is that this is all aligned to your self-image, your internal representation of yourself. What you see on the outside, in the world, is a result of your own self-image. This ties in with the third part of the mindset section, where I'll talk about self-worth, but it's important for you to understand that all of the elements in this part of the book are tied together.

If you have a growth mindset, you'll be seeing what you truly believe you're capable of reflected in your business. However, if you have a fixed mindset you will be struggling with so many disempowering beliefs that you won't have the belief you need in yourself to go after what you really want. Often this is linked to fear. It might be a fear of success, or a fear of failure. The point is, we can all have many fears and these fears will hold us back if we don't learn to disempower them, which empowers us in the process.

When you're scared, you make excuses, or should I say your subconscious makes excuses. This isn't something you'll actively or consciously do, but there will be that little voice inside your mind telling you that it's too hard. Your brain is keeping you firmly in your comfort zone, and the fear of what you might find outside your comfort zone keeps you stuck exactly where you are. Even though we call it a comfort zone, for many of the salon owners I work with this is a highly uncomfortable place.

The trouble is, their subconscious mind has told them that it's more comfortable to stay here than it is to break out of that 'comfort' zone to find out what they're truly capable of or to deal with the issues that really need to be dealt with. This fear of the unknown keeps them pinned into this place that, although it's incredibly uncomfortable, feels safe because it's familiar. There might be some pain or discomfort involved in breaking free and dealing with different issues, but if you take that step, at least there is an opportunity to change. If you just accept where you are and become trapped by this fear then your situation will never improve.

It is important to know your subconscious is always trying to keep you safe, even though it often gets it wrong. It's like a five-year-old child who wants to help you and draws a lovely picture for you on your newly painted wall. You have to train your subconscious in the best way to serve you. Just like if you taught your five-year-old child to only draw the picture on paper, the outcome would be the best result.

TAKE CONTROL: CLARIFY YOUR VISION

When you are trapped in your 'comfort' zone, the fear of the unknown outweighs the fear of where you currently are. What I would like to encourage you to do is make the choice to break free of your uncomfortable 'comfort' zone. This will certainly feel uncomfortable to do and it might even cause you some short-term pain, but when you make a choice and come out the other side, you'll be amazed at what you're capable of.

I always say it's better to endure the short-term pain for the long-term gain than the short-term gain for long-term pain.

Once you make that choice, it's all about taking baby steps towards your broader vision each day. But to be able to have the belief and persistence to take those steps, you need to have a vision in the first place.

Your vision for your salon needs to be incredibly strong. You need to have a purpose and mission.

You need to know who you are and what you want to achieve. This is so important; it's the foundation of everything you'll go on to create because it gives you the drive and belief to deal with situations that might be uncomfortable or painful at the time. You'll tackle them head on because you know that this is for the greater good, to help you achieve that vision and mission of what you want for your salon. You might still be scared, but you won't allow that fear to keep you pinned in your comfort zone any longer.

In some cases this might mean that you lose key members of staff, but it's important to remember that if someone isn't aligned with your mission, then having them in your salon only causes pain in the long run. As I've already mentioned, pain, and a fear of pain, is one of the main reasons why salon owners make poor decisions or avoid making decisions altogether.

In terms of staff problems, it might be that you're scared of losing someone because they might take all the customers with them, which will mean you lose money. Even if losing someone does cause you pain in the short term, if they weren't aligned with your values and weren't working with you to achieve your vision, they would only have caused you greater pain in the future and prevented you from achieving your vision.

It's really important that you stick to your purpose. When you do this, you'll find that you'll be rewarded even from what seem to be negative situations, like a key member of staff leaving your team. I'll share some practical steps that I put in place to help prevent things like customers leaving with a member of staff, later in the book.

For now, I simply want you to understand that there are steps you can take to prevent these pain points. It's part of what I teach in my Salon Jedi Academy. Putting these steps and processes in place puts you in control. When you have control, you can feel more certain that you're not going to lose out and that you can escape from that disempowering mentality. All of a sudden, you won't be scared of someone leaving any more. This all stems from having an incredibly strong purpose.

'I can't give you a higher recommendation than to put yourself in the environment of Caroline Sanderson and learn from her. She understands exactly what you need to do to get you from where you are now to where you want to be.'

-   John Assaraf, 'New York Times' best selling author of 'Innercise', Having It All' and 'The Answer', and world-leading mindset and behaviour expert

LINKING PURPOSE WITH RECRUITMENT

Having a strong purpose and vision is important for a number of reasons, but it can be especially beneficial when it comes to your recruitment process, and anyone you hire should be aligned with your purpose.

In my experience, the members of staff who are causing problems or who leave your salon, do so because they're not aligned with your values and purpose. That doesn't make them bad people and it's not their fault. You both have a different set of values and that's ok, but just know that to reach your salon goals you need people around you who share your values. This isn't about you being better than them or vice versa, it's simply that they aren't in alignment with you and your business. When this is the case, there will always be some conflict over what you're doing, how you're doing it and what your goals are. The clearer you are about your purpose and vision, the easier it will become to find other people who share your values and who will therefore support you on your journey to achieving that vision.
The trouble is that if you're trapped in a fixed mindset, you might be scared of confrontation. You might know that you need to deal with a member of staff, but you're afraid of actually doing something about it. When you behave like this, you often lose control of your salon.

However, when you have a growth mindset, with a firm purpose and vision, you'll know exactly what you want and where you're going. You'll have the inner strength to deal with an issue caused by someone who doesn't share that vision. That's not to say that someone with a growth mindset is perfect, or that they won't have problems. Far from it. However, having a growth mindset allows you to recognise when someone or something is going against your core values and vision and it stops you being scared to deal with it, because your vision is so strong that you aren't going to let this small thing hold you back. You'll develop the attitude that you'll do whatever it ethically takes to achieve your vision, which helps you banish the fear you might have felt about dealing with certain situations before.

FOCUS ON LONG-TERM GAIN

When we make decisions based on short-term gain we look for the quick fix, whether that's having a drink or a smoke, or making a business decision. Within salons, it's common to be short-staffed, but by focusing on short-term gain we make so many recruitment mistakes.

When you're short-staffed, the short-term gain option is to hire someone based on skills alone as quickly as possible. You might have a gut feeling that they're not 100% the right fit for your salon, but they're a great hairdresser with great skills so you'll ignore that voice deep down and hire them because you want to get away from the short-term pain of being short-staffed.

You're not short-staffed any more, but that person you hired turns out to be a nightmare. They cause you long-term pain and, in many cases, will cost your business more money in the long run than they bring in. Trust me, I have definitely made hiring decisions like this!

The alternative is to take that short-term pain for a little bit longer. Accept that you're going to be short-staffed for a while and take the time to recruit someone who is the right fit for your business. When you do this, you might be taking a hit in the short term, but you're creating a better long-term future for your business.

BE PERSISTENT

Persistence is an important element of the growth mindset. It's a big part of what I teach at the Salon Jedi Academy as well. This is all about taking consistent action on a daily basis.

We can all get knocked off track from time to time, that's life. It might throw you a curveball in your personal or work life, but the difference between someone with a growth mindset and a fixed mindset is in how you deal with these curveballs. If you have a growth mindset and something knocks you off track, you'll get back on it again. You are persistent and you will look for solutions to problems rather than focusing on the problem itself.

You are prepared to try different things and if something doesn't work, you'll go back to the drawing board and think about what you can try instead. People with a growth mindset also tend to be more open to change and trying new things.

WHAT YOU CAN ACHIEVE WITH PERSISTENCE

I'd like to tell you a brief story about one woman who joined Salon Jedi. I remember when she first joined that she had a vision, but she just kept getting knocked off track. She had a very small team and she was very short-staffed. She was working a ridiculous amount of hours because she had no choice, but she was trying to balance this with having a young family too. The fact was that she stuck to her goals, she kept her dreambook and was always thinking bigger and focusing on what she wanted to achieve.

Through a great deal of persistence she started to turn things around. She took control of her salon. She put our Salon Jedi systems in place and kept saying 'no, this is how we want to run, these are the systems'. Bit by bit, things improved. Now, she works at London and New York Fashion Week. She's an Aveda ambassador who travels all over the world doing hair shows; she doesn't have to be in the salon any more. Her team runs it and she's able to work on the floor when she wants, but she doesn't need to be there. She's a long way away from where she was when she joined Salon Jedi, as a struggling single parent with young kids who was working ridiculous hours.

What allowed her to turn this around was having that focus and vision, and having the determination every day to keep going, to be persistent, even in the face of setbacks. She knew what she wanted and rather than focusing on the pain she might have experienced in a day, she kept firmly focused on her vision. She developed a support network and reached out for help from mentors too. All of this helped her deal with the emotions of that tough time. The point is she didn't give up.

QUIETING THE NEGATIVE VOICES

As you can see from that example, challenging times are still painful for people with a growth mindset. When I first started turning my business around, the pain was still there. I clearly remember how it felt to walk into my salon and see my staff standing around because there were no clients. Instead of internalising what I saw in a painful way, I would tell myself things like, 'That's okay, I know that it only looks like this because of the way I used to think in the past. This is what I created, but I know my thoughts and the actions I'm taking now are creating a new future.'

I just kept telling myself that my salon wouldn't look like this forever. I kept my vision at the front of my mind. I used to visualise the phone ringing off the hook, clients flooding in through the door into a really busy, noisy and bustling salon. I always kept connected to my future goal and I wrote all my dreams in what I call my dreambook.

This is another key difference between people who are trapped in a fixed mindset and those who have developed a growth mindset: with a growth mindset you are very future focused. As a result, you're able to take the action you need to now, in order to create the future you want to see tomorrow. By focusing on that vision and future, you're able to take a step back from the pain you're experiencing in the here and now and quiet those negative internal voices.

When you're stuck in a fixed mindset you feel the pain in the now. You internalise everything you've created in your world. You feel as though you can't change it. This is why taking that control is so important, because it allows you to change your perspective and with it your future. We all have days that hit us emotionally, but it's our choice whether we 'react' or take the time to think, take a breather and 'respond'.

WHY WORK ON YOUR MINDSET?

Your mindset is your foundation. What you have to ask yourself is would you prefer to stay in pain indefinitely, or are you prepared to have a little more short-term pain to realise long-term gain? This is all about making that commitment. This is the position I want you to be in by the time you've finished this section about mindset. I want you to understand that what you see in your world comes from within you. It's a reflection of your internal circumstances and that's why everything that comes after has to begin here.

Your mindset is the foundation of your business. Your business is a reflection of you as the owner. You have the power to change your thinking, which will positively impact your business.

WHICH MINDSET DO YOU HAVE?

Below are the key traits of the two mindsets I've been talking about in this chapter. Have a look at these summaries, read those stories at the beginning of the chapter and think honestly about where you are with your mindset. There is no right or wrong answer, as long as you know you can change and are prepared to put in the work to do that. You might also be a little bit of both and that's okay too, as long as you are aware.

Fixed mindset

- Problem focused.
- Blaming external circumstances for issues, making excuses.
- Blaming others or shaming yourself (blame turned inwards is shame).
- Saying disempowering statements like, 'This is too hard.'
- Having a lack of direction.
- Focusing energy and attention on things that don't make you feel good.
- Making decisions based on fear.
- Avoiding conflict.
- Trying to control your team.
- Giving up.
- Doing the same things over and over again with the same results.
- Feeling trapped in your comfort zone.
- Feeling stuck and not moving forward.
- Having low emotional energy and losing control of your emotions.

Growth mindset

- Solutions focused.
- Having clear goals.
- Monitoring results.
- Taking full accountability.
- Accepting that problems are part of your journey.
- Asking empowering questions like, 'How can I fix this?'
- Creating clear goals and a vision.

- Focusing energy and attention on your future vision.
- Making decisions based on your goals.
- Taking control.
- Leading your team.
- Being persistent.
- Constantly learning and educating yourself.
- Taking yourself out of your comfort zone.
- Taking daily action and making regular progress.
- Having high emotional energy and accepting and managing your emotions.

I'd like to close this chapter by sharing with you how I made the choice to work towards having a growth mindset, and how I started to take control of my salon and work towards my vision for a brighter future.

My story is one of transformation and I want it to inspire you to realise you can have the success you desire if you choose to...

It was a Wednesday in May 2009 in Inverness in the Scottish Highlands. I could hear the faint sound of a hairdryer coming from the salon floor and the clock ticking as I sat in silence in my tiny salon staff room across from him. I watched as he turned the pages of the report, with his crisp blue suit and short over-gelled hair. The smell of peroxide mixed with his overpowering aftershave, adding to my feeling of nausea.

As I watched him I thought, *You don't look a day over 19, yet you hold my future in your hands.* My tummy was doing backflips, part excitement praying that he was about to deliver the good news I so desperately wanted, and part nervous dread, a deep gut feeling of impending doom.

He looked up at me and, with almost a hint of arrogance, said: 'Miss Sanderson, we can't take on your business to sell it. It just isn't worth it due to the lack of profits over the past few years. I know as a business owner you always think your business is more valuable than it is, but the truth is, it's worthless.'

BOOM. There it was. The news I had been dreading. I wanted to scream at him,

'What do you mean it's worthless? You're telling me my divorce meant nothing? My chronic back pain, that I took painkillers for every two hours for two years meant nothing?!'

The reality was I couldn't speak. I felt numb. 'I'll see myself out Miss Sanderson,' he said in an aloof tone as though I had completely wasted his time.

I'll rewind to explain how I came to be sitting in my staff room, listening to this man telling me that my business was worthless.

In 2009 we were in the middle of a recession. I was eight months pregnant and about to go on maternity leave when my salon manager of four years left work one day never to return. Without notice, she just disappeared to rent a chair across the road, taking my client list with her. She and I were the two main stylists who brought all the money into the salon, alongside a couple of chair rents. Apart from her (and myself) the only other people working for me were two graduate stylists, who helped us on the floor. They were fully qualified, but had never run a busy column before.

As I sat in my staff room that day, all of this and plenty more was going through my head. *How on Earth will the salon survive with two inexperienced stylists, no manager and me off on maternity?*

This wasn't my only problem. I had also gone over the VAT threshold without realising it and owed in excess of £11,000. My fear wasn't restricted to my unfolding salon situation either. I had other pressing worries. I was recently divorced, which was a very painful time, and about to become a single mum to three children. I had no cash in the bank, no savings and I didn't know how I was going to meet payroll that Friday.

The truth was that the recession hit and things were not going well. I had been making every mistake in the salon owner book. That blue suited man was my last hope that day. I hoped he was going to save me and sell my salon so I could get out.

I will never forget sitting in the staff room that day, feeling as though my last hope had been snatched away. *My life is a pile of shit.* I couldn't hold back the tears any longer and, with my head in my hands, I started to cry uncontrollably.

How did it come to this? What have I done wrong? What have I done to deserve this?

These questions kept circling around my mind. More thoughts and voices started to join in. *Caroline, you are useless. You can't make anything work. Caroline, it's not your fault, it's the recession. It's happening all over. Don't be too hard on yourself, everything will be ok. I knew you wouldn't do it Caroline, you are bloody useless. You knew all along you were never going to make a success of it, so I don't know why you're surprised!*

Caroline, listen to your heart. You know you are worth more than this. It's not your fault. You know you can do anything you put your mind to. Then I asked myself one question that changed my life.

Caroline, can you honestly say you have done your best to make a success of your salon?

In that moment, I realised I had not. Initially I felt like a failure for not even giving it my all, but suddenly it was as though a powerful energy force took over. A feeling of pride and power rose inside me, bringing strong determination. At that moment I knew I was not willing to throw in the towel until I had given it my all.

This was my turning point, where the pain felt so great that I had to take action in some direction. There and then I made a decision and a pact with myself: I was going to turn my salon around. With tears drying on my face, I decided I would become number one in my small city, number one in Scotland and, heck, why not number one in the UK?

One of the biggest goals I set myself was to win Scottish Hairdresser of the Year at the British Hairdressing Awards. I felt that this was the biggest accolade I could reach as a milestone that would show it was ME who had made it happen. I also made a pact with myself that I would not only pick myself up and turn my salon around, but that I would share my knowledge with as many other salon owners as I could along the way.

After making that decision, it was time to act. As I was eight months pregnant, I had no choice but to implement systems at lightning speed and train my young graduates to run their columns while I was away. Thankfully I had trained them really well and they were right behind me. As they were both mature graduates, they also had the confidence to use their initiative and follow instruction. This was their chance to shine and they did.

Spending four weeks implementing systems so they knew how to run the salon while I was off was the best time investment I ever made. It allowed me to work ON my business rather than IN it and, after I had my youngest daughter Dixie, I never returned to the salon floor more than one day per week, because the salon was taking in more with me off the floor and working on systems and building my team.

After I returned from my maternity leave and saw how well the salon was running without me on the tools, I took the next steps to grow my business. I looked at the salons that were perceived to be number one in Inverness and decided I would model them. They all had one thing in common: five-star status from the Good Salon Guide.

I took out a loan from the bank to refit the salon, invested in a new computer system and card machine, employed a stylist/receptionist to make sure reception was covered at all times and arranged our first-ever photoshoot. With everything in place, our creative work was published by the Good Salon Guide and the salon featured in our local papers for achieving the five-star rating. I also rebranded our logo to include '5 Star Hair Care' as our tagline.

This was when the business really started to grow. However, I still had one major problem. My salon was situated in a back street location with zero passing trade and I needed more new clients if I was going to grow my salon as I planned. This was when I decided to capture online traffic.

At this stage, I also realised I had been looking at the wrong people to model: if I was only looking at other local salons, I'd only grow to their level. It was time to model the masters, and that meant finding mentors, not in the hairdressing and beauty world but beyond.

My first mentor was Andrew Reynolds, the master of information marketing. He sold all sorts of products online and made millions, getting in front of people who wanted his products with his cash on demand strategy. This is a strategy I still use to this day in my salon. I modelled him to make sure when anyone searched for the highest searched keywords related to salons, my website was number one on Google and that I provided them with exactly what they wanted.

My next mentor was Dan Kennedy, the master of direct response marketing. Once I got in front of prospects and they landed on my site, I needed to know how to write the marketing messages to convert them to clients.

In 2010, I started to master Facebook marketing. No salons were using it at that time and I was the first to create a course for salon owners teaching them how to fill columns with one Facebook post. The results were incredible. I was packing out columns and filling white space all the time, masses of new clients came to our website and Facebook page, and we were the first business in our city to reach 1,000 Facebook fans, which was a huge milestone back then.

There was still one piece of the puzzle missing and that's when I found my mentor John Assaraf. You may have heard of John from the book and film The Secret. He is a New York Times best-selling author and CEO of Neuro Gym, which applies scientifically proven methods and technologies for helping people expand their mental and emotional power. As a firm believer in the law of attraction, I came across John's Winning the Game of Money programmes and set to work on my mindset as well as the practical elements I needed to grow my business.

By 2011, two years to the day after sobbing in the staff room, we were the first INAA Scottish Hair Salon of the Year, as well as winning two other awards. By 2012 I had expanded into a salon that was double the size of my original premises to accommodate over 2,000 new clients that year.

By 2013, we had taken an extra £131,000 in 12 months and trebled the salon business. I also became the first female to win Creative Head's Most Wanted Business Thinker and we were crowned as the best salon business in the whole of the UK. This award is open to any salon business across the UK, so that was my tick moment of being awarded number one in the UK as part of my goals.

In 2015, I was finally crowned Scottish Hairdresser of the Year at the British Hairdressing Awards, at the very first time of being a finalist; achieving the benchmark I had set myself to know I'd reached the top goal purely by my own creation.

I have gone from a back street chair rental salon owner on the brink of bankruptcy to a multi-award-winning salon entrepreneur with multiple streams of income, an international speaker and, by the time you read this, a published author with a goal of becoming a best-selling author. I believe so strongly that if I can do it in my industry, anyone can do it in theirs; it's just a case of following the same steps I took.

CHAPTER 2

SUPER SELF-MASTERY

In the last chapter I talked about how what you see in the world around you is a reflection of your internal world. This chapter is all about how you can become a master of your mindset and emotions to allow that internal world to manifest what you want to see in the external world.

Many people find that they keep hitting a glass ceiling. The same problems are holding them back again and again. There are several obstacles that can hold you back and prevent you from breaking through that self-imposed glass ceiling. These include your emotions, your limiting beliefs, your perception of your self-worth and not having the right skill set. In this chapter, I'm going to explain how you can master each of these areas.

LIMITING BELIEFS

All of the experiences you have in your life, good and bad, shape your internal beliefs. Our brains take a snapshot of our past experiences and use those to form the basis of the beliefs we hold today. That's great if your brain creates empowering beliefs for you, but all too often our beliefs are disempowering. These disempowering beliefs can make us feel as though we're not good enough or we're not worthy, which means we either try something once and give up when it doesn't work, or we don't try at all. These are the limiting beliefs that we need to master.

This is challenging, because often these limiting beliefs extend back to experiences we had as children. The way I like to think of the brain is that it's like a computer, with an operating system. Your beliefs are an important part of that operating system as they're what you've used to programme your brain. But, much like in an actual computer, your internal operating system can be changed.

However, often we find that our brains are resistant to change, especially around our core beliefs. This is because your brain protects what it knows, which is the current operating system. It's a bit like it has its own version of antivirus software in there that's protecting its programming. As a result, your brain only shows you the things that are related to and support your beliefs, which just install those beliefs even more deeply. Your brain shows you an image of the world that is based on your internal beliefs. It's what I talked about in the last chapter, about seeing what you have on the inside reflected back on the outside.

For example, if you believe that you're only worthy of taking a certain income, let's say £20,000 a year, you might make decisions that cap you at this level without even realising. I know some salon owners out there don't even pay themselves that much and they really struggle. What I'm asking you to do now is to think of a limiting belief and explore where it comes from. If you're struggling and struggling, working really hard and barely making any money, I suggest you think about why that might be. Do you always find that, just as you're starting to make progress and your salon is starting to get busier, that something happens to pull you backwards? Maybe it's a stylist going on maternity leave, or a couple of stylists or therapists leaving to rent chairs. All of a sudden you're back to square one.

As I've said already in this part of the book, it isn't that you'll be making conscious decisions that prevent you from making more money, but your subconscious beliefs, this operating system in your brain, will make you see the world according to those beliefs, instead of allowing you to see the opportunities that can help you override them.

UPGRADING YOUR PROGRAMMING

As I've also said, just like a computer, you can upgrade your programming. This is what you need to do if you're going to progress. You need to upgrade your limiting beliefs. The first step to doing that is to be aware of them.

Listen very closely to your internal narrative. What are you telling yourself? Do you find yourself saying you're not good at something? Or making sweeping statements like 'it's impossible to find good staff'? You need to catch yourself when you're talking to yourself in a disempowering way. It's only by doing this that we can master ourselves.

In your mind, when you say a phrase like 'it's impossible to find good staff' you're creating a statement of fact for yourself. You're making that your reality because that's what you're going to see. I see salon owners saying this all the time and then they wonder why they can't find good staff. It's because their brain is focusing on everything it sees in the world that supports that belief.

This particular example isn't even necessarily just a limiting self belief. It's actually one that I see perpetuated across the whole hairdressing industry. I regularly hear people telling me that it's impossible to find good, trained staff. Yes, there are issues within the hairdressing industry in terms of not enough young, trained staff coming through, and others leaving the industry or going self-employed, but while that might sometimes make it harder, that doesn't make it impossible. It's also something that we, as an industry, need to work on. From a personal perspective, however, you have to start by working on your own belief system.

When I hear this kind of limiting belief being given a voice, I always ask, 'But is it possible?' I'm not saying that you'll be flooded with CVs of good quality, well-trained staff, but is it possible to find the right stylist for that position?

When I ask this question, I'm often met with a host of excuses, like 'it's only a small town' or 'no one good ever sticks around', but they're not thinking of all the possibilities. They're trapped in that fixed mindset with this limiting belief. To free yourself from this limiting belief, start believing that it's possible that someone with the skills you're looking for could move back to your town. Instead of something being impossible, you're choosing to believe that it is possible.

FINDING MY SALON MANAGER

To show you just what can happen when you shift your beliefs, I'm going to tell you about how I found my salon manager. She is without a doubt the best salon manager I have ever had.

Many years ago, I was falling into this belief that it's impossible to find good staff. One day I decided that I wasn't going to buy into this belief any more. I did a simple exercise that transformed my belief. I wrote down all the possibilities of how I could attract this amazing manager to my salon. I thought it could be someone who was moving back to the area. Maybe they had left to travel the world and now they were coming home. Or maybe they had moved away for a relationship and now they'd decided they wanted to move back to Inverness. They might have decided they wanted to settle down and raise a family in the Highlands. I came up with a whole list of possibilities.

Then I visualised receiving CVs. Sure enough, CVs started to arrive at the salon. Now, some of those CVs were from people who were totally unsuitable for the position, so I revisited the exercise and made sure I was very clear. I told myself that I always get CVs from people who are perfect for the position. To cut a long story short, my current salon manager applied and she's brilliant.

She was a big part of how we made our record-breaking results at my salon in 2019. For example, in one week, she did £6,500 – and that's not selling expensive electricals or hair extensions. That was what she took, by herself, in just one week. She was smashing it. I still only have a small salon with a small team, but we get exceptional results and I put this down to mindset. Not only mine, but the team's too. I've encouraged them to believe in themselves and to open themselves up to what's possible.

Self-mastery is really all about having that awareness and being mindful of when you are talking to yourself in a disempowering way. Once you catch that, you can start to create new beliefs and they will pay off. This is about creating new habits, which I'll talk more about a little later in this chapter. But the thing with creating new habits is that there is an uncomfortable period when you're creating that new habit. What you have to remember is that it's no more uncomfortable than what you're experiencing when you're struggling. It's the fact that it's new and uncomfortable that prevents a lot of people from creating that new habit.

BREAK THE CYCLE

This comes back to what I discussed in the previous chapter, about finding the strength to break free from your comfort zone. As I said, for many people their comfort zone is actually an incredibly uncomfortable place. They have become so familiar with struggling, that they find it hard to break the cycle.

Remember your brain's operating system? It's trying to keep you in this familiar place, a place where you're safe and secure. By keeping you in your 'comfort' zone your brain believes it's keeping you safe and conserving energy. That means you'll often feel as though it's too much effort or energy to break free from this 'comfort' zone. What I'm telling you is that you can override this programming, but to do that you have to break the cycle and step into that uncomfortable feeling. Tell yourself that you're going to keep doing that because you know you're creating a new habit, which in the long term will bring you benefits.

Again, this all ties in with what I talked about in the first chapter, about being persistent and accepting some short-term pain at times to realise that long-term gain.

LIMITING BELIEFS DON'T END WITH SUCCESS

Again it's important to know that even if you are successful in your business, that doesn't necessarily mean that limiting beliefs aren't still holding you back. To the outside world, someone might look like they're doing incredibly well. They might have multiple salons, some of them might be really big, but they may still be working very hard and struggling for not enough reward.

Your salon can be turning over hundreds of thousands of pounds a year, but if you're only paying yourself £25,000 and you're having to work incredibly hard for that money, it's time to start asking yourself what the point is and explore why you're not earning more. Do you have a limiting belief where you only believe you're worth a set amount a year? It's your money thermostat. Do you find that no matter how much busier you get and grow, you still keep earning around the same amount of money?

No one is immune from holding these limiting beliefs. If you're working really hard and have three salons that are doing well, but then you take on another salon somewhere else that's losing money, it's just cancelling out the hard work you're putting in. We can always work on our mindset and it's not a process that stops as you become more successful.

CHUNK IT DOWN TO THE RIDICULOUS

I talked in the first chapter about having a big picture, a big vision, in your mind that gives you the strength and belief to take yourself out of your comfort zone, create new habits and do what's necessary to move forward.

The trouble is, even if you've got the big picture in your mind, if it's too big then you just don't believe it's possible. What I want you to do is chunk your big picture down to the ridiculous. When I'm working with people, I tell them to set a goal and often I can tell that they're writing it with no belief whatsoever.

For example, their goal might be that they are going to do an extra £150,000 at their salon this year. To help them realise that it's possible, I get them to chunk it down to the ridiculous. When we start doing that, there's always a moment when I see the light bulb switching on, because they realise that it is possible. That's when their belief starts to grow, and what often happens among my clients is that the figure they want to achieve increases, because they realise how possible it is.

For instance, it might be something as simple as asking a salon owner if they think they can get all of their stylists or therapists to do one treatment in the morning and one in the afternoon, because that's all that's needed. Let's say they have six stylists and each of them is doing that many treatments per day. When you look at it like this, add up what that means in a week and then multiply it by the six of them over the year, they might find that it'll hit their goal. That's the light-bulb moment. What seemed huge suddenly seems very achievable, all because they've chunked it down to this ridiculously small level. That's how you get the brain shift and find the belief to go for those big goals.

I usually recommend that people look three years ahead. Once you know your timescale, you can take an average of how much extra you need to make each year to achieve that. You break it down by the number of staff you have, how many days of the week you're open and so on. You chunk it down, chunk it down and chunk it down. All of a sudden you might get to a point where you realise that all of your staff just need to take an extra £100 a week, for example. If you're struggling, you might feel as though you've been trying to get them to do this for years, but that's where I can help. I want you to first believe that it's possible; then I want you to see what you need to do to achieve your goal. After that, we'll work on the details of how you achieve that goal and what you can do to increase sales, for instance.

If we take this example of needing your staff to each take an extra £100 a week, one of my recommendations would be to create a package that provides loads of value to clients and that costs £99. That means each member of staff just needs to sell one package a week. By giving people the tools, I can see that belief start to kick in. It takes time to change your brain's operating system and to break free of these limiting beliefs, but by breaking everything down into manageable steps with clear actions, you can do it.

Gradually, momentum will start to build and your results will accelerate. You've got to think of this process a little bit like climbing a ladder. You can't go from the bottom rung straight to the top, you have to go step by step.

What you have to watch is that as momentum builds, you don't lose your sense of purpose. I'll talk more about how you can manage that growth and maintain it as momentum builds, in the maintenance part of the book.

STAY CALM: MASTER YOUR EMOTIONS

As well as maintaining your focus you have to stay calm. This is especially true when you start to see your salon moving in the right direction. I see people getting a bit too excited, or allowing their ego to take over. There's nothing wrong with having drive and ambition, and the ego acting as a driver for that, but you need to ensure you remain in control of your emotions. You still need to make decisions in a calm and practical manner, rather than making emotional decisions.

For example, you might decide you want to open a second salon and you go and view a bigger salon. It's great that you have that ambition. However, what you have to do is take the emotion out of your decision to acquire another salon.

I've looked at many acquisitions over the years and I've never gone through with any of them because I don't make my decisions based on emotion. I've looked at salons and thought, 'Oh my God, I want this'; but I have my price, I know my figures and I know it's not worth any more than that. I'm not prepared to pay over the odds to satisfy my ego. The reason being that when you have to work ten times as hard to make a return on that investment, to me it's just not worth it. I've certainly lost a couple of acquisitions as a result of my approach, but that's fine.

When I'm coaching salon owners who are looking at other premises, I always recommend they talk to me first before they make an offer on another salon. I just want to ask them some calm, clear questions to make sure they're not buying emotionally. I want to see that they've thought it through properly, that they understand the location, why the current owner is selling it, what the staff are like and, of course, the figures and client lists. I'm not trying to burst their bubble, because if there's something you really believe in and you want it, you should go for it. What I want them to do is take the time and have the awareness to see if they're making decisions based on emotions. It's important to take that step back and look at what you've got. I want to encourage my students to be calm and rational enough to make a decision that considers the whole picture.

It's important to have this clarity about your decisions because that can also stop you making a decision based on fear. When you're motivated by fear, you tend to make the wrong decision, whereas when you look at a situation objectively and calmly, you see it differently and you often make a better decision. You have to be responsive, rather than reactive.

LOOK FOR LEVERAGE

Sometimes when you're in the thick of things it can be difficult to see opportunities for leverage within your business. I have no doubt that somebody else could walk into my business and see areas of leverage that I've missed, but learning to find leverage and maximise it will really help you to grow your salon.

Leveraging your time is an important part of this. Taking myself out of the salon allowed me to spend more time working on the business and growing it. This actually highlights another limiting belief that I encounter, which is that you've got to be at your salon to grow it. I'm proof that this isn't true.

As long as you have the right mindset, put the right systems in place, develop the right culture and hire the right people into your salon, you don't need to be there. You can leverage your time. You want to avoid being the person who's trying to do absolutely everything and instead focus on what you're best at. If you love running your column, doing the hairdressing and interacting with your clients, that's fine; but if you don't want to do all the other things within your business, you need to find someone who can.

Someone has to be managing the business, driving the sales targets and so on. Do they have to be at the salon in person? That's arguable. Managing the business and driving sales virtually is just as legitimate, you just need to make sure you have someone who is taking responsibility for that.

It's really difficult for one person to be super passionate about every aspect of the whole business and to be the key driver for every area. It's not a realistic expectation for anyone.

Think about the job description: you're looking for someone who will run a full column, be the manager, do the marketing for the salon, spend some time on front of house, do a bit of cleaning and also be the bookkeeper and do admin.

You wouldn't expect anybody else to do all of that in one job, but these are the expectations that we put on ourselves as salon owners. These expectations become self-imposed shackles that hold us back. When you learn to release a bit of control, you will see that you can leverage your business and achieve much greater things.

I was guilty of being too controlling at one stage. I was forced to let go because I was pregnant and going on maternity leave and, once I did, I realised that my salon could work without me.

SET BOUNDARIES

When you start to release control and allow others to step in and take on various aspects of your business, it's essential that you set boundaries for yourself and your team. Without these, you won't break free of the mental shackles you've placed on yourself.

One example is getting off the floor as a salon owner. When I made the decision that I was getting off the floor completely, I set very clear boundaries. I couldn't count the number of times that I could have gone back on the floor, and it's tempting because when you're short-staffed and you're busy you could be losing a couple of grand a week; but I never went back on the salon floor. I knew that if I did, it would be like I was saying to the team that I was there. I would be making a rod for my own back, because then whenever a stylist was off sick, I'd be the person they called to come in. By going back on the salon floor after deciding to step away from it, it would almost have been as though I was giving them permission to take time off, because I would always pick it up for them. So very early on, I decided that I would never do that.

I also set very clear boundaries around my role at the salon. For instance, when I took my front of house manager on I was still working one day a week on the floor. My manager isn't a hairdresser, her job title is Client Manager, but on the day I was working, some of the staff would still come up to me and ask me a question. I would always respond with, 'Okay, ask Carla.' I wouldn't even try to answer their question. This might happen a few times, which is what does happen when you're creating a new habit. After a few times of coming up to me and receiving the response, 'Ask Carla', all I'd have to do is look at them and they'd say, 'I'll ask Carla.' I kept doing that until eventually they all stopped asking me.

Everyone knows now that Carla is the manager of the salon and nobody asks me anything any more. I'm just not there in that capacity. To some extent it's become a passive income for me, because although I enjoy doing the marketing, I have leveraged that income stream to allow me to step away from it.

DISCIPLINE OR REGRET?

There's a quote that I heard from my mentor John Assaraf and it's one that comes to mind often: *'You either pay the price of discipline or you pay the price of regret. Discipline weighs ounces, regret weighs tonnes.'*

In terms of your mindset, it might be having the discipline to bear that short-term pain, as I've already mentioned. Or it might be having the discipline to form new habits.

Changing a habit isn't easy and it takes a lot of discipline. It might take 30 days, 60 days, even 90 days or a year, depending on how long that habit has taken to form and how deeply rooted it is. What you have to remember is that, even if it takes a year and a lot of discipline to change a habit, you will then spend the next 30 to 40 years without that habit that was holding you back and instead with one that drives you forwards.

I'm certainly not perfect. I still have limiting beliefs and I am a work in progress, just like anybody else. You don't suddenly become perfect in all the areas of your life. We all have multiple limiting beliefs and it takes time to change them. This book certainly isn't about being perfect. But it is about having that awareness that there are areas where you could improve and that you have beliefs that are holding you back.

Another question from my mentor John that I like to ask people is, 'Are you interested or are you committed?' If you are just interested, you won't do what it takes, whereas if you're committed you'll do whatever it takes. In my presentations I often say that I'm interested in being a size 10, but I'm not committed so I don't do what it takes in terms of exercising or prioritising my diet to get there.

If I was committed to that as a goal, it would be my priority every day, rather than work and the projects that I'm doing, but it's not that high up in my hierarchy of values; although this can change. I can tell you that I'm committed to growing my business, helping others and empowering people. I'm absolutely committed to my mission. That's easy for me as it's highest in my hierarchy of values.

EXERCISE

UNDERSTANDING WHAT YOUR VALUES ARE

There's a simple exercise you can do to help you understand what your inner values are, and how these might be holding you back. Listed below are six values, and I'd like you to put these in order of priority for you. There is no right or wrong answer to this. You will know what the most important value is because it's the thing that you work towards every day easily without having to be prompted to do so. We all know health is important, but if you are overweight and not exercising then health is not your highest value. Our highest values are the things we are most committed to.

- Career
- Family
- Health
- Money
- Social
- Wealth

Once you've put those values in order of priority, look at what you have in your top three. What you need to understand is that anything near the bottom of your list will be put behind the values that are higher up. So, if you put money at the bottom of your list and it stays there, you will never do what it takes to make more money. Most of the people I work with will tell me they want to make more money, so the key to helping you change your priorities is to link money to one of the values you have higher up your list of priorities. Let's say that family is at number one, in which case you can look at how you can link money to your family. Having more money could allow you to afford private healthcare, or it could mean you can have more experiences with your family or travel with them. Doing this can help you question your beliefs around money.

WHAT AFFECTS YOUR PERFORMANCE?

How we feel has a lot to do with how we behave and our inner value system. It's all linked to your energy because your results will track the energy levels that you have. This is about identifying the specific things that cause a drop in your energy levels and make you feel low. This is important because when you feel low you don't perform at your best, and you either don't take action or you take weak actions because your energy is weak.

We have our highest energy and flow when we are working on our highest values. We often get knocked off track when we are doing tasks we don't value that are keeping us from doing what we love. This is why outsourcing is key when growing. Get rid of the £10 an hour tasks and pay someone to do them for you while you do what you do best; because when you are doing what you love, you are in the flow and you will stay on a higher vibration of higher energy and get better results.

EXERCISE

WHAT ARE YOUR TRIGGERS FOR POOR PERFORMANCE?

I'd like you to take a few minutes now to write down five things that trigger you to not perform at your best. It could be anything, from eating too much sugar, to not getting enough sleep.

1. _____

2. _____

3. _____

4. _____

5. _____

Sometimes it can take you a while to realise what those triggers are for you. For example, I know that sugar drops my energy levels, so cutting out sugar, or even just reducing it, has a positive effect on my performance. I also know paperwork and bookkeeping trigger me, so I outsource these along with many other tasks, which leaves a happier, higher-performing me.

Your triggers could be completely different. It might be skipping your exercise, not going for a walk at lunchtime and getting some fresh air, procrastinating, not getting enough sleep, or not meditating. Whatever triggers you identify, think about whether you can reduce or eliminate them from your life.

What I often find is that there are many people out there who are struggling to keep going and who think they can't achieve what they want to, but a lot of this comes down to their lifestyle and the fact that they are doing so many things that trigger them to have low energy.

Once you have identified your triggers, you can look at what daily rituals you can introduce to empower you. Make these daily rituals your new habits. Flip the five triggers you've listed in that exercise and see whether you can either reduce them or stop them completely. Often the steps you need to take can be very simple. One of mine is to listen to meditation audiobooks when I'm walking. Once you know what lifts you up, make a conscious effort to do more of that and less of the things that trigger you.

This is a very simple idea and these are very small steps, but they are ones that many people just don't take. They don't form these positive daily rituals and that means they don't see their performance improve.

This exercise is about listing five triggers and flipping them. If you know sugar triggers you, flip it to reduce or eliminate sugar. If paperwork triggers you, set out to outsource it and so on. Use the exercise below to flip your five triggers and then list five things that you know lift you. When you do this, you end up with ten actions that I call your super self-help bible.

EXERCISE

Flip your triggers. How can you turn the triggers you listed above into positive actions?

1.

2.

3.

4.

5.

Now list five things that you know lift you.

1.

2.

3.

4.

5.

If you create these daily rituals of little things that lift you up and flip your triggers, you'll start to feel better and you'll start to perform better. That's when you start to see results. The key is sticking to these daily rituals. Once you feel better and start to see those results, it can be easy to forget to do those daily rituals. When that happens, you'll slide backwards again. It's very important to be consistent and not to stop your daily rituals just because you are feeling better. They need to become habits.

LEARN TO LOVE YOURSELF

When you equip yourself with the right kinds of tools to lift you up in your life, you're practising self-love. A big part of creating the right mindset is learning to love yourself and understanding that it's okay to do that and to put yourself first.

I often meet people who feel guilty for giving themselves time for their daily rituals, but it's important that you set aside time to do the things that help you perform at your best. This is essential to developing your inner self-worth.

The more we love ourselves, and live in our highest values, the more certain we are of ourselves and the more clarity we have, the less we care about being judged and failing. Developing this sense of self-worth helps eliminate your fear of what other people might think or your fear of failure. This is when you will tell yourself 'I'm worthy of this' and you'll believe it. It's about saying, *'I'm worthy of changing my life. I want to change my life. I love myself enough that I'm going to commit to this.'*

Having this self-worth gives you the confidence to try things and to think big.

EXERCISE

HOW GOOD IS YOUR RELATIONSHIP WITH YOURSELF?

Before we move into the final chapter on mindset, I'd like you to complete this short exercise.

Score yourself on a scale of 0 to 10 on how good of a relationship you have with yourself. You'd put this at 0 if you really hate yourself, while you'd put this at 10 if you love yourself.

Really think about how much of a friend you are to yourself when you're deciding on that score. Often we tell ourselves horrible things and would never talk to other people the way we talk to ourselves.

Think about whether you're disempowering yourself, or whether you're lifting yourself up like you would with a friend or family member. If you realise that you're beating yourself up a lot, sit with that awareness for a moment and carry that awareness with you so that you can quiet the negative self-talk in your mind.

This is certainly something that I had to change in myself. What I realised in doing so is that the more sure you become of who you are, what you're doing, what your purpose is and what journey you're on, the more you run your business with love rather than fear.

The more I'm at peace with myself and the more I love myself, the less challenging problems seem to be and the easier it is to deal with those curveballs that life throws at you. It really is a different way of living. The more we love ourselves, the more we back ourselves and the more we know that the universe has got our back, the more we'll push ourselves out of our comfort zones and work towards our vision. None of this is about external forces at work – it's all about you and what you can achieve yourself.

'I know without her guidance and support I would not have been able to achieve my goals or even believe I could have such goals to reach. I can honestly say that Caroline has made the most positive impact in my life and her generosity and guidance and belief in me means I cannot fail.'

- ***Carla Zebrowski, Salon Managing Director & Salon Jedi Coach***

CHAPTER 3

PRIDE AND PROFITS

What I mean by pride is self-worth. You've probably heard the expression, 'Your self-worth equals your net worth.' This is all about feeling worthy of receiving.

We all have beliefs around money and what we're worthy of earning. What you feel worthy of earning will depend on the people you surround yourself with, what your parents earned and what past experiences you've got around money. All of these elements combine to create our beliefs and install those as part of our brain's programming. In doing so, we create our own money thermostat and define what we think we're worth.

I can remember as a kid thinking that being a millionaire or having a lot of money was something that happened to other people. I didn't think for a second that someone like me could go after a goal like that, which is completely crazy.

This all comes back to your self-worth. Often this starts to get shaped very early in our lives. Whether you're brought up around a lot of money or around scarcity, whatever you know from a young age becomes your internal representation of money. If you're brought up around scarcity, you might form the belief that money is hard to come by, for example.

It's important to understand how this internal representation affects what you achieve. You might realise that you want to make more money and decide that this is a goal you're going to go after, but if your internal representation of what you're worth financially doesn't match your desired new level of income, then you won't get it. Instead what happens is that you sabotage it. This isn't deliberate. Remember how we talked about the subconscious nature of limiting beliefs? This is just how your brain keeps you in line with your internal reality, or money thermostat. It's making sure your outer reality reflects what's going on internally.

This means that unless you change that inner thermostat, you won't be able to get to the next level because you will just keep sabotaging yourself. It might be that you make a little bit more money, but all of a sudden you lose it again because the car breaks down or something goes wrong. Life will just go on like this until you alter your internal thermostat. Feeling as though money is hard to come by, having to work extremely hard to make money, all of these things are linked back to your self-worth.

You need to stop and ask yourself why you have to slog your guts out and work your fingers to the bone just to get by. When you start to examine this, you'll almost always discover it comes back to a limiting belief you were unaware of.

What I teach my students is that, if you want to turn your money thermostat right up, to get it to a really high level, you have to break everything down into manageable steps. Chunk it down to the ridiculous. Let's say you're earning £20,000 a year and you want to be earning £200,000 a year. The difference in those figures is too great. It seems too far off and that makes it seem too hard to achieve. That's when you turn back to those limiting beliefs and start telling yourself that you're not good enough to create that, or you can't do it, or it seems too hard. Often it's because you don't know HOW and I always say the how doesn't matter. Once you believe it you will be shown the way. Returning to those limiting beliefs disempowers you instead of empowering you to make positive changes and work towards resetting your thermostat to a much higher level.

STARTING TO BELIEVE IN WHAT'S POSSIBLE

As I mentioned in Chapter 2, what you need to do is chunk your big vision down to the ridiculous. What I've found is that when you have enough self-worth to just move up one level, not a huge jump but a small step in the right direction, then you can make gradual adjustments to your internal money thermostat that will stick.

Let's say you start by aiming to increase your earnings from £20,000 a year to £30,000. Once you get to £30,000 you have to decide what level you're comfortable aiming for next. Maybe you aim for £40,000, and then £50,000. Once you get there, do you feel comfortable increasing your earnings to £100,000 or is that too big of a step? If it is, go up in smaller increments and maybe aim for £65,000.

Those are just arbitrary figures to give you an example, but the point is that you're lifting your self-worth up little by little to help you believe that the bigger picture is possible. When you have such strong internal programming, it is very difficult to have that self-belief to see yourself earning £200,000 a year when now you're only earning £20,000. However, if you go little by little then it's much easier for your mind to adjust. If you spend time around people who are just one step above you too, it's much easier to believe in what's possible.

In 2019 when I set out on my mission to reach and teach 1,500 salon owners through events, at my first event of the year we took £12,000. At our final event a year later, we took £78,000. I would never have thought that possible at my first event, but step by step the events grew.

You still need to have a big picture or a long-term vision, like I mentioned in Chapter 1, and it's essential that you're not only connected to that big picture but that you believe it's possible. Your desire might be to earn £100,000 a year. You don't need to know how to do it right now, you just need to be connected to that desire and believe that it's possible. These small steps I'm talking about are a way to reprogramme your mind, to change your internal thermostat, to make sure that you have that strong belief in your ability to achieve that big picture.

BIG VISION, SMALL STEPS

You can't compare yourself to someone who's already where you want to be. You have to remember that even if they have a chain of salons, with great websites and their marketing and branding spot on, it wasn't always like that. They had to start somewhere. Rather than focusing on what they have (and what you don't), work backwards. Look at your big-picture goal and decide what halfway between where you are now and where you ultimately want to be will look like. Think about what that feels like. Could you see yourself doing that halfway step, does that make sense? Yes, then brilliant. Work towards that halfway step, believe that you can reach that halfway step, and always have that next step in mind.

This is about realising what it will take to bring your big picture to life. There will be processes, procedures and systems in place that you need to set up. You need to be taking consistent and continuous action towards making that happen.

WORK WITH MENTORS TO HELP YOU RESET YOUR THERMOSTAT

Breaking your vision into bite-sized chunks is just one thing you can do. Spending time with people who are just above you on the ladder is another good way to help you develop your self-worth and belief. Working with a mentor can also be a useful way to learn and start giving you that belief in what's possible.

Investing in yourself is important and if you surround yourself with like-minded people who have a strong sense of self-worth, it will help you to believe more in yourself. You constantly need to be growing, developing and challenging yourself to push out of your comfort zone. If you don't make changes and just continue to spend time with the same people you always have, you'll just reinforce the self-beliefs you have now rather than forming new ones that can help you achieve your vision.

Investing in your self-development or your business is a good example of how you can start to break out of your comfort zone. You need to view investment as a way of taking that next step on the ladder. It can be scary at first, especially if you're spending a lot of money, but this comes back to the idea that you have to spend money to make money. You need to believe in yourself in order to have the courage to make that investment. When you do that, spending that money is no longer a risk, it's an investment.

Money, or more specifically a sense of a lack of money, is often a limiting factor in people investing in themselves; but if you're going to climb that ladder, you need to believe in investing in your journey. An investment is completely different to a cost, but when you're paralysed with fear and you're spending that money from a place of fear because you're hoping this will be some kind of magic wand, you're viewing it as a cost. This fear stems from not having faith in yourself and not believing that you're worth it and can achieve your vision.

In my experience, most people are very unaware and this is where mindfulness around money, as well as mindfulness around business, is particularly important. Mindfulness just means being aware. When people talk about having a mindful attitude towards money, all that really means is that they have an awareness about money. Developing that awareness takes a little bit of digging. You have to look back at your past and do some exercises to really examine where your limiting beliefs around money have come from.

Some of you might know that you have limiting beliefs, because you can see the results in your external world, but not know the root cause of those beliefs and therefore not know how to fix them and change them. That's what I'm here to help with.

FOCUS ON ABUNDANCE, NOT SCARCITY

When it comes to dealing with your limiting beliefs around money, it's the same as dealing with any other limiting beliefs. You can retrain your brain. Just as I mentioned earlier in the book, where you are right now is the result of your brain's operating system and you can upgrade this by doing things like 'innercising' and retraining your brain.

One of the most important elements of this is being aware of what the issue is and understanding where it comes from. Often the biggest problem that people have when it comes to money is that they've created scarcity in their reality. When you do this, it becomes a perpetual cycle and it is difficult to override, although certainly not impossible.

There are only two fundamental core human fears at the reptilian brain level: fear of losing that which we seek (e.g. being the predator and NOT getting your prey, which leads to starvation) and fear of being the prey (getting eaten by a predator). To bring this example to money, a fear of not getting the money you seek and a fear of losing the money you have. So, when you are striving to make more money or hold on to money from a place of fear, you receive more lack. When you focus on your purpose and goals and move towards your goals with clarity and being of great service to others, with no fears, you reach your goals.

This feeling of scarcity can come from a number of places. It might be that your business hit a little slump and you focused all your attention and energy on this scarcity, which created fear around it. This fear locks you into a cycle where you focus on the scarcity instead of on the abundance. In time, even a successful business that was doing really well before it hit a little blip can start to struggle more and more. This is because whatever you put your focus and energy into is what expands in your life.

Or it could be that you start your business from a place of scarcity because you don't understand investment. It's this idea I talked about earlier, that you have to spend money to make money, but for some people that is a scary concept.

The way I like to explain it is that investing in a business is like building a snowman. You can't build a snowman without a small snowball to start you off. As you roll it, it gets bigger and bigger and bigger, but you need that little snowball to grow in the first place. Many people open a business and are scared of investing. They aren't even giving their business a chance to grow because they aren't starting with that small snowball. From the beginning, they're in a mindset of scarcity. Often they'll have bought their business with a bare minimum and will be working on a shoestring budget. As a result, they're always looking to spend the bare minimum of what they've worked really hard for.

The problem with this approach is that they aren't thinking about what they can be comfortable with and what they can afford to spend money on, such as training or a new website. They don't look at how much they need to borrow to make the business work and grow. They are stuck on that shoestring, in that scarcity mindset. What happens is that, even if they do well for a while, they don't put enough aside, and then as soon as there's a bit of a downturn, they don't have the foundation they need to feel secure. They start in a scarcity mindset and it just gets worse and worse.

I have met people who have had their business for ten years and they still don't get paid. That's crazy, but that's the reality. They're working every hour they can, but by this stage it's become an emotional issue. They're scared of letting go of their business, they're scared of being judged and they're scared of failure. They are completely stuck because they can't escape from that scarcity mindset.

If you've read any of those scenarios and feel that they are familiar, what do you have to do? Someone once said that thinking the right way is the hardest thing that a man or woman has to do. When you're seeing this reality of scarcity and lack, you have to change your thinking. You have to tell yourself that everything you're seeing right now is the result of everything you've thought and seen up until this point. If you want to change what you're seeing, you have to change your thoughts and focus. You have to shift your focus not to what you don't have now, but to what you desire.

Rather than looking at a shortage of money or a shortage of clients, you have to visualise your phone ringing off the hook. You have to visualise money flooding into your till. Visualise how your salon reception will look and sound when it's busy with customers and stylists and therapists chatting, hairdryers going. Think back to the two stories I told you right at the start of Chapter 1 and how Jenny, the salon owner with the growth mindset, would visualise her future.

I'm not saying this is easy. I have been in this situation myself and I have used these visualisations. Believing in those visualisations and that future is probably one of the hardest things I've ever had to do. When I was standing in an empty salon, I would keep telling myself that although it was real, it was just a reflection of everything I'd done until that point. I kept telling myself that everything I was doing now was creating my new future.

One trick I used, and it might sound a little daft, is that as I was paying bills, I would draw smiley faces on the cheques. I became a happy taxpayer. Instead of focusing on what was going out, I was focusing on what was coming in.

I see this time and again. People spend too much time focusing on their bills and outgoings. They put a lot of negative energy, feeling and thought into that. Then, before they know it, there's another unexpected bill, followed by another, and they're wondering why this is their reality. It's because this scarcity, this lack, is what they are giving their focus, attention and energy to.

You will have to go through a period of time where you flip this in your mind. Even when your outer reality is far from what you want, you need to flip it in your mind to make yourself feel good about it. Know that this is part of the process of changing and stay committed to your visualisations. Make sure that every day you're connecting with what you do want, rather than what you don't want. Putting in this commitment to form new habits is essential. These are not only new ways of being, but new ways of feeling. This is all part of the process of reprogramming your operating system.

I also used to play the 'What if?' game. What if I find a way to master something new that brings in new customers? What if this is the right training course for me? What if I won awards? I would always focus on a positive 'What if?'

Even though it's such a simple thought, it's very difficult to change. But I would urge you to be an actor or actress because sometimes you just have to pretend for long enough and then what you want, all that abundance, starts to be reflected in your outer world.

DON'T RESIST THE UPS AND DOWNS

Just because you focus on abundance, that doesn't mean you'll never experience scarcity. Life ebbs and flows, sometimes bad things happen, but that is just part of life. It's the universal law of polarity. We don't live in a one-sided universe, we live in a perfectly balanced universe where we get equal amounts of highs and lows. In every high we can find a low and in every low we can find a high if we look for it.

The trick is knowing when to go with the flow. It's a bit like trying to swim against the current of the outgoing tide. Rather than fighting that current, conserve your energy, because you know that the tide will turn and flood in again. Don't try to resist this ebb and flow. Go with it and do the best that you can in the challenging periods.

Often if you conserve your energy when the tide is going out, you can go even further when the tide is coming in because you have the energy for that extra push. You can build momentum and go a little bit further each time the tide comes in for you, and that means you won't drift out as far each time the tide goes out.

You have to be aware of these shifts and make it a habit to keep working on yourself. You'll always have things you can be working on and it's important that this is what you focus on. If you don't, it's all too easy to drift away into the everyday niggles and issues, and before you know it, you've been dragged a long way offshore.

CREATE DAILY CLARITY

One of the reasons why people can drift off with these issues is that they don't have enough daily clarity. I would recommend giving yourself three critical things to do each day, for instance, and making sure you do them really well. Put yourself into the mood you want to be in. Be active in your day.

Too many people become a passenger in their day. They just react to whatever shows up, rather than responding from a calm emotional state. They open themselves up to distraction after distraction and then they wonder why they get knocked off track. This ties back to the difference between those with a fixed mindset and those with a growth mindset.

When you have a fixed mindset, you're a passenger in your day who only sees the problems, whereas when you have a growth mindset you're the driver who focuses on finding your way around the obstacles in your path. If you don't fill your day with your high-priority actions, your time will be stolen by others. You will end up scrolling social media, answering emails and being highly distracted.

BECOME AWARE OF YOUR PATTERNS

When you feel like every day is Groundhog Day, you fall into this negative pattern and it can be very hard to break out. All of us can fall back into patterns and habits, often without even realising we're doing it.

That might be a pattern of speaking to yourself in a negative way, or a pattern of behaving in a negative way. When you still have a negative internal representation of yourself, you can fall back into those patterns of behaviour very easily. Most people aren't aware of their patterns, or how they reinforce them.

The first step to breaking these patterns is to become aware of them. At least if you have that awareness you can change it or flip it. Also remember we have an equal amount of good days and bad. The goal is not for every day to be perfect, but to see perfection in every day no matter what is going on. This perfect balance is just like us. There is no one who is perfect all the time and the pursuit of this perfection will only bring you more unhappiness.

HOW TO START BREAKING FREE OF BAD PATTERNS

To start developing that awareness, which will help you break free from these negative patterns, you need to look at the reality of where you are right now. What is your financial situation? What is your team like? Are you mostly seeing great results at your salon? Do you rise to challenges? Are you solution focused? Be honest about whether you're struggling financially and are in a place of pain.

The first step is taking accountability for your external reality and understanding that this has come from you. Once you accept this and take responsibility, you need to commit to changing. This all starts with you. You have to change how you feel about yourself, you have to change your self-worth. This is what pride and profits is all about. If you don't have the self-worth to stand in your own beliefs and core values at the salon and to deal with the issues you face, then that's what is creating the problems. You really have to work on building your self-worth and that means committing to this on a daily basis. It all comes back to you. Remember the exercise at the end of Chapter 2, where I asked you to assess your relationship with yourself? What was the outcome of that exercise for you? Hopefully it's helping you to see where you need to work on your relationship with yourself to help you build that self-worth.

WHAT CAN YOU EXPECT FROM WORKING ON YOUR RELATIONSHIP WITH YOURSELF?

When you start to improve your relationship with yourself, there are a few things that you'll begin to notice. In a general sense, you'll start to feel more empowered and you'll have greater belief that you can achieve your goals.

This starts with a small flicker and then builds and builds until it becomes something more substantial, where you have that self-worth, you're able to dream big, you are confident in dealing with issues and solving problems to create a better business. You'll be more aligned with what you create and you'll be prepared to take more risks to achieve your vision. All of this goes hand in hand. You'll naturally start to see the benefits of having an improved relationship with yourself.

As you learn to upgrade your mindset, you're laying the foundations that you need to create that vision and turn it into your reality. Improving your relationship with yourself, increasing your self-worth and upgrading your mindset is very much a foundation. But if you do this and nothing else, you won't make millions and your life won't necessarily change substantially.

All of what I've talked about in this first part of the book is a foundation. Once you're building pride and profits, you are laying a strong foundation and from here you can start doing all the other things that I'll talk to you about in the coming chapters. You have to upgrade your mindset first, and once you have that foundation in place, you can upgrade your skill set. That's when everything will start to fall into place.

Without having this sense of self-worth, you won't achieve the success you're striving for. It might be that you already have empowering beliefs and a strong sense of self-worth without being aware of it, in which case you may have less work to do in this area than others, but that doesn't mean that you can't improve on what you already have.

Although this chapter has focused on money and generating profits, that's not to say this will be the only limiting belief that is holding you back or making you unhappy. There could be many things that you'll need to work on internally to create the vision of the world you want to see. I've used money as the example in this book because it's an area that many of my students want to, and often need to, work on.

> *'Caroline has a unique way of inspiring the audience and catching their imagination with her mindful training, at the end of the course it left them feeling like they could take on the world. I wouldn't hesitate to recommend Caroline and her team no matter what type of business you're involved with.'*
>
> - *Barry Stephens, Managing Director, Mutu Ltd, Chairman Fellowship of British Hairdressing*

My job, whether you're reading this book or on one of my courses, is to help you believe in yourself. I want to inspire you to take those first steps. I want you to learn about my story and see that I'm not special. If I can do this, so can you. What I want you to take away from this first part of the book is an awareness of the importance of your mindset, and an awareness that you need to do work inside yourself, on your inner world, if you want to get the best results from your business and in your life in general. All of the knowledge and actions that come in the following chapters will undoubtedly help you to grow your business, but I can't stress enough the importance of getting your mindset right first and laying that strong and stable foundation.

CASE STUDY
CHRIS & EMMA

We're Chris and Emma Simmons. We own Salon 54 in Thirsk, North Yorkshire, which we've been running since 2001. We've certainly experienced challenging times; in fact, the first 13 years that we had our salon were stressful and very hard work. We've been working with Caroline since 2014, which at the time of writing is six years. In those six years, we've turned our salon around with Caroline's help and we'd like to share our story with you.

2014

Every day we'd wake up and not want to go to work. We never knew what stress we'd find when we got there, but we just knew there would be some form of stress or drama every day. All we could see in our salon was what we lacked. We struggled to make enough money to pay our bills. We always noticed what our staff weren't doing. We felt angry inside and as though we were always on the back foot. We saw all of the negative aspects of our business, but we didn't know how to fix them.

Things got worse and worse. We felt like we were only just keeping our heads above water and every day felt like a constant struggle. We carried around this dread and fear from the moment we woke up until the moment we came home, but even at the end of the day we couldn't relax because we'd be thinking about what had gone wrong that day, or what might go wrong the following day. We were stuck in a very negative cycle.

We felt completely trapped and, because both of us worked at the salon, if we just closed it then both of us would be without an income (not that we were making a lot from the salon at this stage). It was a stressful and scary place to be and neither of us looked forward to going to our own salon in the morning.

The catalyst for change

One day in 2014 we received a phone call from our bank manager, who told us that we needed to put more money into our account because we didn't have enough to pay our staff's wages that week. We were already well over our overdraft limit and we had a feeling of complete panic. We were scrambling around the salon trying to find whatever money we could. We emptied the float from the till,

Chris emptied his pockets, I emptied my handbag. We were grabbing whatever we could find down to the last penny. We just needed enough money to pay the staff's wages. Obviously at this point we weren't paying ourselves. This was when we realised we needed to do something. We were reaching the end of the road.

We felt that our only option was to change how the salon operated and go to a rent-a-chair model, which would mean all our staff would be self-employed and we wouldn't have to worry about paying their wages. How much they earned would be down to them, not us. From the outside, it looked like it would take all the stress away from us and that was all that we wanted. It felt like the only option left without just closing the salon.

But neither of us knew how rent-a-chair salons really operated, so we decided to go to an industry event, Salon Smart. Our hope was that we could meet some people there who ran their business in this way and that we could learn how to do that ourselves. Then Caroline came on stage.

As she talked about her story, how she'd almost lost her salon and how she'd turned it around, we realised that she was the person who could help us. She wasn't just another professional speaker, she was someone who had been there and come through it. She understood our situation. We needed to talk to her. The problem was, it seemed like most of the salon owners at the event felt the same! She was surrounded by a sea of people after she came off the stage and we couldn't get anywhere near her. We went back to our hotel and emailed her, because she had said she'd take 100 salon owners on to help them with their mindset. We wanted to be among those 100 people, but given how many others clearly wanted her help, we didn't think we'd make the cut.

On the train on the way home, we were both feeling deflated. But then Chris's phone went ping. We had an email from Caroline. We could join the group. We couldn't stop smiling. That was the day our lives changed.

Upgrading our mindset

Emma

Caroline started by giving us work to do on our mindset before she even mentioned the business. She gave us a book to read about how you thought about money and where your beliefs around money came from. I decided that

I was going to do everything she said, because that was the only way I was going to get through it. Chris was more sceptical. He couldn't believe someone would offer something for nothing and his initial reaction to the mindset work was, 'What a load of mumbo jumbo!' But I had told myself I'd do whatever Caroline said, so I persevered and started to notice positive changes.

Chris

The mindset work has always been challenging for me. I was a very negative person and I didn't realise how negative I was until I started doing work on my mindset! Initially I couldn't believe that Emma was buying into that stuff, but I started to see a change in her and it made me think twice. Then I started to do some of the exercises and learn more about it. I've always struggled to read a book, so I found an audio version and listened to that. The more I did, the better I got and the happier I felt. Now I'm always listening to audiobooks and podcasts while I'm doing other bits and pieces.

What changed?

The most important change was that we started seeing what was good about our salon. We stopped focusing on the negatives and started seeing all the positives. Our change in mindset rubbed off on our team too.

We're sure that most salon owners can relate to having issues between staff, where the people on their team bitch and moan about each other, the owners, the salon, the customers and anything else. Before we started working with Caroline, our team was very negative, but when we started to become more positive, so did they.

Now we have an amazing team who are happy and fun-loving. They might not all be the best of friends, but they all get on really well and they have each other's backs. There are no nasty comments or snide remarks. Everyone gets on, works well together and nobody moans about anyone else. Our staff also don't take sick days.

Caroline also gave us the confidence to enter awards, which we had never really done before. That first year, we entered one of the biggest hairdressing awards in the country and became finalists. Since then, we've been finalists and winners of over 100 awards.

Financially, the turnaround has been amazing. When we went to Salon Smart, we were overdrawn by between £10,000–£11,000. Six years later, we have around £90,000 sitting in our business account. In 2019, we turned over £204,000 and we had to go up a VAT bracket. In 2020, we are on track to turn over £309,000, despite the global pandemic!

For us, the VAT bill is a really important one. We always used to struggle to pay our VAT bill and every year it would wipe us out and make us miserable. Now we're really happy when our VAT bill comes because we know that if that bill is high, then we've made a lot of money.

Of course, the mindset work isn't all that we've done. We've worked on marketing and all the other areas you're going to read about next. But we honestly believe that if we hadn't started by changing our mindset, everything else we have done wouldn't have worked. We had to change our outlook because we were negative and that ricocheted through everybody in our team, as well as our customers.

When you are positive, that also ricochets through your team. They become more positive, you all earn more money, your customers feel happier. You have to put yourself in the right headspace for everything else you're doing to have a positive knock-on effect through the whole business.

We make sure we reward our staff for their hard work and we have always been honest with them about how the business is performing, because it means they'll understand when we need them to work that little bit harder. We also work on our team's mindset, because this helps to keep their lives stress free and makes them happier, which only has a positive effect on the salon.

Everything started by changing our mindset

Without changing our mindset, we wouldn't have achieved half the results that we have. This shift in mindset was so big for us that it made all the difference to every area of the business. Changing our mindset made everything else in the business fit and work. Without it, we wouldn't have had the persistence or commitment to tweak, change and adapt other elements of the business. For example, six years ago if we'd run a marketing campaign and it hadn't worked as well as we'd hoped, we would have just given up. Now, we'll tweak it and see what we can do to improve it. We don't give up.

Although we might have been a little sceptical at first, we can see exactly why Caroline made us start with our mindset, before we even looked at any numbers or figures. It really is the core of how everything else comes into play.

ARE YOU LIKE CHRIS & EMMA? IF YOU'D LIKE TO KNOW IF YOU HAVE ANY LIMITING BELIEFS HOLDING YOU BACK, YOU CAN BOOK A FREE BREAKTHROUGH DISCOVERY CALL. SCAN THE QR CODE BELOW USING YOUR MOBILE PHONE'S CAMERA AND SELECT THE TIME THAT WORKS FOR YOU.

This breakthrough call is to look inside your business to see how to improve profits, scalability and leverage, and to identify any limiting beliefs holding you back.

We will help you discover what is not working in your salon business and plan how to scale up and reach your dream profits, even while getting off the tools if you wish.

PART 2

MARKETING

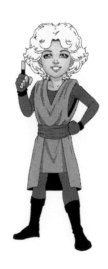

Marketing is the key to building any business. It doesn't matter how amazing you are or how skilled you are at what you do if people don't know about you. You need to get your message in front of your ideal customers and set yourself apart.

Your mindset is the foundation, the core of your business, and that all starts with you. Marketing is about your clients. Once you've got a strong foundation, it's time to start attracting clients to your business because you need them to be able to perform your work.

A lot of salon owners don't do any marketing, or the marketing that they do is very minimal and they take a scattergun approach where they throw a lot of things out there and just see what happens.

In this part of the book, I'm going to explain the five steps you need to take to master your marketing and help you become more focused in your marketing activity.

CHAPTER 4

REVEAL

There are two parts to reveal. The first is revealing who you are, what drives you and what your niche is, and the second is revealing your ideal client avatar. A significant part of the work for this first aspect of reveal, in terms of finding out who you really are and what drives you, will happen when you're working on your mindset.

A lot of the work I do with my students involves really drilling down into what their passions are, understanding what drives them and, from this, revealing their purpose. Think for a moment about what you are best at. Ask yourself what you want to be known for. Use this understanding and knowledge of yourself to create your purpose.

> *'It has been a pleasure working with you on your "Online Brand Assessment". It gave me a deeper appreciation and understanding of your thoughts, process, goals and challenges. I was very impressed with your background, business ideas, intelligence, experience, and friendly personality.'*
>
> - **Howard Lim, Fortune 500, President of How Creative**

FIND YOUR NICHE

An important part of this element of reveal is finding your niche. Once you've found your passion and your purpose you will know what you want to deliver and you can carve out your niche. Many of the salon owners I work with are terrified of carving out their niche because they worry that if they do this, and only market to their ideal client avatar within this niche, they'll repel other customers. But what you have to remember is that not all clients are equal and that means not all clients will be your ideal clients.

It might seem difficult to get your head around, but it's okay to repel customers if they aren't the kind of customers you're looking for. This is what marketing is all about. You should be marketing to attract your ideal customers and to repel the ones that don't fit into this avatar. Aside from anything else, this will mean you don't waste your marketing budget. You have to be smart with your marketing budget and leverage it to get the best return that you possibly can.

I'll come back to how you can carve out the right niche for your salon a little later in this chapter.

WHO IS YOUR IDEAL CLIENT?

Revealing your ideal client avatar is the second part of reveal. To do this well, you need to get that first part, where you reveal your true self, nailed down. This isn't just about defining your ideal client avatar, but thinking about where you will find them.

Many of the salons I work with will initially tell me that they'll take any client that's breathing, but if you want to take your business to the next level it's essential that you know exactly the type of customers that you want to work with and who will want your services. For example, if you want to sell your hair extensions, it's no good putting that marketing in front of a bald man. That might be an obvious example, but failing to think about who your ideal client is, is one of the biggest marketing mistakes I see salon owners making.

DEFINING YOUR IDEAL CLIENT AVATAR

Let's say that your salon wants premium clients. How might that avatar look?

My ideal avatar is female. She's a working professional who has money and who values premium services. She is willing to pay for these premium services and wants the best service. She appreciates quality.

If you're going to effectively target the people who fall under this avatar, you need to know as much as possible about them. Answer the following questions for your ideal client avatar:

- What age group are they in?
- What professions will they typically work in?
- What TV do they watch?
- What newspapers and/or magazines do they read?
- What social media networks do they use?
- What events do they go to?
- What hobbies do they have?
- What kind of car do they drive?

You can even give your avatar a name if you want to really step into the shoes of your avatar. The more you can learn about them, the better. You can carry out research, do polls and speak to the clients who come into your salon who fall under your ideal client avatar. Find out as much about their needs and desires as you can. Learn what drives them and what problems in their lives you can solve.

YOUR IDEAL AVATAR WON'T BE YOUR ONLY CLIENTS

Even if you come up with an incredibly clear ideal client avatar, that doesn't mean they are the only people you're going to attract. Not everyone who walks through your salon door is going to be a 34-year-old HR officer who watches Love Island, reads Hello!, drives an Audi and spends £1,000 a year on their hair.

The point of your avatar is to focus your marketing. When you're writing marketing content, you're writing it with them in mind. The avatar you create won't describe every single client you get, but if you really target your marketing by speaking to your ideal client avatar, you'll find that your clients generally share similar traits.

Not everyone who falls under your ideal client avatar will see your messaging either, but what you have to think is that if the ones who do start shouting about how amazing your salon is and telling their friends, word will spread. It will have a knock-on effect.

HOW TO TARGET YOUR IDEAL CLIENT AVATAR

If you've decided that you want to target a premium ideal client avatar, start by thinking about how they want to feel. They probably want to feel as though they matter. They are willing to pay for premium services to feel significant. If that's the case, make sure you put a premium price tag on your services.

Another mistake I see salon owners making is targeting those premium clients but heavily discounting their services. I call it 'death by discounting', because this attracts the wrong kinds of customers to your salon. Don't get me wrong, I'm not against discounts when they are presented in the right way with a strategy behind them, such as if it's to attract a new customer, or if a customer is paying for services in advance, or if they are buying a bundle and spending a large amount in one go; but too many salon owners discount everything because they see other salons doing the same and think they have to follow suit. The first lesson to take away from this is that if you want premium clients, you need to charge premium prices and your service had better be premium to match.

You also need to think carefully about how your marketing materials look. If you're going after premium clients but you're using cheap marketing materials and messages like everyone else, do you think they'll look twice at your salon and services? No, because they won't think that you're what they're looking for.

A premium client is looking for value, a good experience, quality and something different. They will value your skills and that means that you need to value your skills and position yourself to showcase them. Your marketing material needs to look the part. Remember that you're not trying to target everyone.

DO YOU DO DRY CUTS?

I remember when I first opened my salon, we'd get the odd walk-in. They might be a pensioner who came in to ask if we did dry cuts. I would always say, 'Sorry, we don't do dry cuts.' These people would always leave because they would look at the price of a wet cut and take their business elsewhere.

That's fine. The people looking for dry cuts were not, and are not, my ideal client avatar. Once you have revealed your ideal client avatar, you have to be okay with the fact that this means you will repel those other people who aren't willing to pay for, or who don't have the budget to spend on, premium services. That's okay. The more you focus on attracting your ideal client avatar, the more of them you will see walk through your door.

WHERE DO YOUR IDEAL CLIENTS HANG OUT?

When you're building up a profile of your ideal client avatar, it's very important that you consider which social media platforms they use and what magazines or other publications they read, because this is where you're going to want to target your marketing.

These days the majority of marketing is done online, so you need to know which platforms your ideal clients spend the most time on. Remember that just because you have a platform that you prefer to use, whether that's Facebook, Instagram or Twitter, that doesn't mean your preferred platform will be the same as your ideal clients' preferred platform. Find out where your ideal clients spend the majority of their time, and you need to go to them. You can use other platforms as well, but make sure that your main focus is on where you're most likely to find those ideal clients.

I would recommend choosing your top three marketing platforms for your strategy. That doesn't mean you won't use others, but you will focus most of your attention and energy on those top three. To make that list, you have to work out where most of your customers come from. For my salon, our top three marketing strategies are Google, Facebook and referrals. It's important that you don't just focus all of your activity on one platform, because if something happens to that platform you will still have customers coming in from other sources.

DON'T BE AFRAID OF BEING NICHE

As I said earlier in this chapter, many people are terrified of carving out a niche. Let me explain why it's so important to find your niche and do everything you can to slot into it.

Let's say that your ideal client avatar is busy, professional women. These types of people broadly fall into two categories when it comes to the likes of hairdressing and beauty. Some will want to have a day to themselves where they can get pampered at the salon. They'll want to take time out of their busy schedule to relax and unwind, as well as having their hair cut or getting a treatment or whatever else you can offer.

Then there are the other busy professionals who still want a premium service. They still want the best, but they want it at speed. They want convenience and they don't want to take a whole day just to get their hair cut or coloured. As a salon, you can't easily target both of these clients with the same marketing messages and you can't provide the service they are each looking for in the same space. You can still target both of these avatars, but you have to adjust your marketing and service accordingly.

For the clients who value speed and quality, you could set up an area in your salon that provides premium express services. For the clients who enjoy pampering, you can designate another part of your salon to be a relaxing and calm environment where you can take your time to deliver that service. You need your ideal client avatar to match what you offer. You can't be all things to all people.

The next trick is to create two separate marketing messages, one for each of these ideal client avatars. Avoid falling into the trap of trying to market to both avatars at the same time. If you do this, you'll dilute your message and then it isn't as strong. That means you won't stand out and you're likely to miss out on capturing your ideal clients.

What you can do, however, is create a strong and clear marketing campaign for your premium express offering, and a separate marketing campaign for your premium pampering offering. These marketing campaigns will be worded differently and targeted differently to ensure you stand out to your ideal clients.

Another similar example, and I have tried to do this myself too, is when salons rent out a bit of space to a beautician who's a sole trader offering these beauty treatments. The problem is, when you do this, you're never going to stand a chance against a beauty salon that is purely a beauty salon.

If you're going to add beauty services at your salon, then either you or the person who's driving it needs to be fully passionate about it. Just like you live and breathe a passion for your salon, you need to have this same passion for beauty, because customers can tell and the ones who really value those beauty services will go somewhere that specialises in them. This goes the same for beauty salons who rent a hair area in their beauty salon.

HOW REVEALING YOUR NICHE AND IDEAL CLIENT AVATAR HELPS YOUR ADVERTISING

I'd like to share a practical example with you to illustrate the importance of being very specific about your niche and who your ideal client avatar is.

I'm going to talk about Facebook advertising for this example. In my experience, what a lot of people do is create a Facebook ad, boost the post and just see what happens. They don't target their advertising and then they wonder why someone who lives a hundred miles away, who's never going to be their ideal customer, engages with the post. However, Facebook allows you to run highly targeted ads and that means you can put your adverts in front of your ideal clients.

Let's imagine that you're running a Facebook advert for wedding hair or makeup. On Facebook, you can target people who are recently engaged. You can specify that you want your advert to be put in front of women who have got engaged in the last three months. You could write your ad to say: 'Recently got engaged? Do you realise that this is the best time to make a plan with your salon to do your wedding hair and makeup?'

Then you could run another, highly targeted, advert for women who got engaged six to 12 months ago. That advert text might be something like: 'Been engaged 12 months? It's time to plan your wedding hair.' Being very specific in your targeting is a much better use of your marketing budget than running either more generic adverts, or specific adverts without making sure the right people will see them.

As soon as you have revealed your niche and your ideal client avatar, you have a much better chance of attracting those ideal clients to your salon, and you'll spend your marketing budget in a much more efficient way.

YOU CAN CREATE MORE THAN ONE AVATAR

You don't just have to create one avatar for your ideal client. You might have more than one goal. So while you're targeting these premium clients, for example, you might also want to get known within the industry. The way to go about that will be different to how you attract those premium clients, so create another avatar.

Your second avatar could therefore be your peers, other hairdressers, therapists or beauticians, so that you can target them not to win them as customers, but to build a name for yourself and grow your profile within the industry.

CHAPTER 5

REEL

Reel is about hooking your ideal clients and reeling them in. In marketing, it's your message that is the hook and line. You have to make sure that your message is a match to your ideal client avatar.

If you think back to the example that I gave you in the previous chapter, where you're running a highly targeted Facebook advert for someone who has got engaged in the last three months, your hook would be the headline: 'Recently got engaged? Now's the time to start planning your wedding hair!'

In that example, you're directly speaking to your client avatar, you're calling them out. Another example might be: 'Exhausted entrepreneur? Come and relax in our luxury spa.'

In the second example, you're calling out your avatar's pain. Are they stressed? Are they exhausted? Tell them how your services can help them with that in the headline. Hook them with the headline, then start to reel them in with some more information that will increase their interest.

You also need to touch on your clients' desires. If they're recently engaged, they're going to want the perfect wedding hair and beauty. Make sure your advert shows them how you can do that for them.

DIFFERENT HEADLINES FOR DIFFERENT PLATFORMS

When you're running Facebook adverts, you have to remember that people will be scrolling and you need to grab their attention. This is interruption marketing, so whatever you put in your advert has to stand out. The headline is just one part of that. You can include emojis as well as text if that fits with your message and branding. You should also use an image or video to help attract attention. It's important that your advert relates to that first thing that people see though. If you post an advert with a completely unrelated image, just as a way of grabbing attention, people will feel it's not authentic and they're likely to move on.

On Google, however, you might take a different approach to your headline and focus more on someone's pain point. If someone is searching on Google, it's often because they have a pain point and they're looking for a solution. If you can tap into that you're more likely to attract attention for the right reasons.

DON'T FORGET THE CALL TO ACTION

One of the main mistakes that I see people making with their marketing is failing to have a call to action. If you're giving someone a solution to their problem, or you're telling someone how you can give them exactly what they're looking for, you need to make sure that there's a way for them to access that. You have to make it easy for people to contact you. Give them a clear call to action, whether that's the option to book an appointment online or to call to book an appointment.

Each bit of your marketing is to get your customers to do the next bit.

THE AIDA MODEL FOR MARKETING

What I've just described falls under the AIDA model for marketing:

- Attention: you have to grab their attention.
- Interest: you have to provide them with more information that interests them and keeps them reading.
- Desire: you want them to have a desire to learn more and to use your services.
- Action: this interest and desire leads them to your call to action.

Your call to action needs to be very clear and very specific.

CREATING A WEBSITE THAT WORKS

All too often I go on a salon's website and it's just like a business card. There's no information on there about how you're going to make your customers feel, how you're going to serve them or even an obvious way for them to contact you. The salon isn't asking for an email address or asking someone to book a consultation call. They're just providing the bare minimum.

What you have to remember is that no one is going to book an expensive treatment through a website like that. People want to know more, they want to chat to you. Give them that option, make it very clear what they should do next and make it very easy for them to take that next step.

If you have managed to get to number one on Google or another search engine for a specific search term, such as 'hairdressers in [your town]', people will be landing on your website, but they will just bounce off if you don't look the part and give them very clear next steps to get in touch with you or book an appointment.

If you're targeting premium clients, your website needs to match their expectations. If it looks homemade and there's no call to action, people will make a judgement very quickly and then they'll leave. If you want to run a premium salon, your branding has to match that. If you've done the work of getting your website near the top of the Google results page, don't waste it!

Your website is the first impression of your brand and even if you're the best at what you do and you're brilliant, if your website isn't good and doesn't make a good first impression, you're never going to get that customer to take the next step and come to your salon.

TIPS FOR WRITING YOUR MARKETING MESSAGES

The most important thing to remember with marketing is that each step is designed to get your customers to take the next step.

There are some key things to bear in mind when you're writing your marketing materials:

- Who you're writing your message for; that's your ideal client avatar.
- Use the rules of AIDA when you're writing your marketing messages (Attention, Interest, Desire, call to Action).
- Your headline is what hooks people. Take time to craft this and get it right. A very simplistic example might be: 'Professionally done hair without the wait.' Or that headline could be for a 60-minute makeover package. You're taking away the 'pain' of having to spend a long time at the salon, or having to wait for a treatment, and you're giving them what they desire, which is beautiful hair.

There are lots of ways in which you can approach this, but what you're aiming for with your headline is to show someone a benefit while taking away a pain point.

Other things to consider using in an advert include:

- Risk reversal: this is where you offer a guarantee.
- Testimonials or social proof.
- Positioning: this might include sharing expertise, accreditations or awards.

A NOTE ON RISK REVERSAL

As you know, most salons will fix hair, nails, etc. for free if someone isn't happy with it, but there is very little mentioned about this in most salons' marketing. That means if you advertise that you're offering a money-back guarantee on a particular treatment, or maybe on a new stylist or therapist, it will really stand out to your customers.

In my experience, many salon owners are too scared to offer a money-back guarantee because they're worried that customers will take advantage of it, but most people won't do that. More often than not they will give you the chance to try and fix something before you have to give them their money back. Let's imagine that you ran a money-back guarantee on a particular treatment and you got ten new customers as a result, and just one wasn't happy and asked for their money back – you've still got nine new, happy customers due to your guarantee. You have to treat the one you refunded as a marketing cost. This comes back to your mindset and focusing on the positives rather than the negatives.

THE 'WHAT'S IN IT FOR ME?' RULE

'What's in it for me?' (WIIFM) is really important to bear in mind when you're writing any marketing message. Your clients are only interested in what's in it for them. A common mistake I see on many salon websites is that they're talking about themselves without mentioning the customer and what they can do for them.

Your customers want to know what you can do for them. This doesn't mean you shouldn't talk about the fact that you've won awards, or that your team are trained in a particular way, it just means you should think about how you can use that positioning while telling your customers how that benefits them.

For example: 'We're an award-winning salon and our team do XYZ training so that you know you're in safe hands with our experienced stylists.'

That still tells your customers you've won awards, it still tells them that you're highly trained, but what you've done with that sentence is make that information relevant to them.

A top tip is to read aloud any piece of marketing material that you write. Pay attention to how many times it says 'Me', 'I', 'We' as opposed to 'You', 'Your', 'You'll'. That can be a great eye-opener and show if you're not focusing on your customers enough.

I'm not saying that you should never use 'Me', 'I' or 'We', of course sometimes you have to, but make sure that you always relate this back to a benefit for the customer.

'I have made an EXTRA £10,963.50 since joining Salon Jedi 14 weeks ago. Not bad, eh? To say I'm on my own plus one new stylist I had to take on since starting Salon Jedi? I'm really pleased.'

-   *Clare Pearson, Ash Hair*

USING THE RIGHT MARKETING LANGUAGE

The language to use for marketing messages tends to be conversational, especially on social media, but you still need to adapt your language for different platforms. For example, on social media you might want to use emojis in your marketing messages, but you wouldn't use emojis if you were writing an article on LinkedIn.

It's also important to remember that even within platforms, you may need to adapt your language and messaging. Facebook marketing is different to Messenger marketing, for instance. In Messenger, you're talking directly to one customer, which means you can't make it sound like an offer or a deal, you have to show your value in a chatty way, whereas in a Facebook advert you can be much more explicit that you're providing a specific offer.

CHAPTER 6

REVENUE

There are different parts to revenue but what I'd like to focus on is pricing for profits. This is one of the most common areas where salon owners fall down. The reason they get their pricing wrong is because they do the following exercise – and I know this because I did it myself. Before they open their business, many salon owners call around the other salons in their area to find out what they're charging. They find the average and then, often, they'll price themselves a little above the average because they're confident in what they do, but they very rarely price themselves near the top, or consider charging more than the top-priced salon in their area.

If you're aiming for premium clients, as I've talked about earlier in this part of the book, you have to use premium prices. Premium clients are willing to pay a premium, so your business model is fundamentally flawed if you're only pricing yourself just above average.

> *'This week I will use packages again to get more business through Facebook. I know that I will get another £1,270 on packages. 90% of clients went for the highest-priced option, there was a lower-priced option. Prices were £40 to £60 more than usual, so I am making double on every cut and blow dry by calling them Ultimate Redesign for the cost of shampoo & conditioner.'*
>
> - **Jenny Curry, Sensational Hair**

The other reason why this approach to pricing doesn't work is that there are too many variable factors in running a business. By pricing in this way, you're not pricing based on profitability, because you aren't thinking about a multitude of other factors that will affect how much money your salon will make.

These factors include: Do you have overheads? Do you own the building you're in, are you renting the space, or are you mobile? If you do have a bricks-and-mortar building, do you pay rates on it? Do you get rate relief? What size is it? What's your rent? What's the maintenance on the building that you have? Do you employ staff and, if so, how much do you pay them? What about the cost of your stock suppliers? There are so many factors that come into play.

Another common problem I encounter among salon owners is that they don't increase their prices as those variables become more expensive. If your rent goes up, or your staffing costs go up, your prices need to go up too. All too often, salon owners will hold the same prices for years because they are too scared to raise them. That means that every year they become less and less profitable.

What I find very interesting is that if you were selling a physical product, you would base your pricing on how much it costs to make or buy that product, to ship it and to get it to your customers. You would never sell your products for a loss. Whereas in the service industry, I often encounter people who pluck their prices from the sky and that means they're selling their services at a loss.

They can work all the hours God sends and it won't matter how busy they get or how many stylists or therapists they have working in their salon, because if they haven't priced for profits, they aren't going to be profitable.

Often salon owners will think that they need to get more money in the till, so they'll get a new team member, but, again, if that team member isn't profitable then it's costing you to have them there. Obviously when someone first starts they're not going to be as profitable as someone who's worked in your business for years, but your aim should be to get them to break even from day one.

At my salon, that's always our aim with a new member of staff and we have a 12-week plan whenever a new stylist starts so that we know exactly how much they need to take from day one to make sure they break even and it's not costing us money. What we do is treat each individual stylist as a business, in effect.

My point is that you need to understand your numbers, otherwise your salon is never going to make you a profit and earn you money, no matter how good you are or how hard you work.

DON'T FOCUS TOO MUCH ON YOUR BREAKEVEN

In my experience, the majority of salon owners don't have a good enough understanding of their numbers, but every now and then I'll work with a salon where the owner tells me they watch their figures, they know exactly what their breakeven is and their main target is to make breakeven each week.

To show why this isn't where your focus should be, I'll tell you about a salon I worked with recently as part of a transformation day, where I go into a business, look at the accounts, the figures, the team stats, the KPIs (key performance indicators) and everything else. In this particular salon, the person who was responsible for driving the business forward just kept telling me that she made sure that every week they hit their breakeven. I asked, 'What do you get each week?' and her reply was, 'We break even.'

This comes back to what I talked about in the mindset part of this book. Whatever you give your focus and attention to is what you get more of. In this case, the salon was always breaking even, but the owner never gave any thought to turnover or profits. That meant there were no targets there for profits on top of that, so the salon was stuck just breaking even.

YOU'VE ONLY GOT ONE PIE

You only have one pie and that pie will add up to 100%. Let's say you're aiming for 20% net profits. The other 80% of your pie will be made up of wage costs, stock, rent and so on. If you overspend in any of those areas, there's only one place that extra can come from and that's your net profit, unless you cut back in another area.

I've even worked with salons that are not only eating into their net profits, but they're spending beyond them. That means they're operating at minus figures and barely even making their breakeven, let alone making a profit. I've worked with salon owners who aren't really paying themselves, which means they often aren't even earning the minimum wage. They're living hand-to-mouth, grabbing bits and pieces of cash where they can, but that's not really living. When you look at how many hours they're working and compare that to what they get out of the business, you quickly see that it's not much at all.

PUTTING THE FOCUS ON YOUR GOALS

I said earlier that you shouldn't place too much focus on your breakeven, but you still need to be aware of it. You need to work out your average monthly or weekly expenses for your salon. Then you need to look at your goals and what percentage of that pie you want to be net profits. Once you know all of those figures, you can work out what you should be charging per hour.

This means you're creating your pricing based not only on what your expenses are, but also on how much you want to make, which is a big difference.

At my academy, we are very goal focused when it comes to revenue. One of the first things I get my students to do is decide what their goal is. They answer the question, 'How much do I want to make?' That becomes their main focus. As I mentioned in the mindset part of the book, some salon owners find this very challenging because they are so used to thinking within the confines of what they're earning now that they struggle to see beyond that.

What I encourage all my students to do, and what I encourage you to do, is to think bigger. Don't just think about what you think you can do, think about what you want to do. How much do you want to earn? If you could choose a figure to be earning right now, what would that be? Write it down and from there you can reverse engineer it. I'll talk more about reverse engineering and managing your figures in Chapter 14.

What normally happens when salon owners see their three-year goal broken down into very small levels is that it doesn't seem as big as they first thought. This comes back to what I talked about in Chapter 2, where I said that you need to chunk your goals down to the ridiculous. This starts to trigger the belief that you can achieve your goal and even open more salons in the future.

Before you consider opening another salon, however, I would stress the importance of making sure you leverage your current salon fully before you move on. Leverage what you have and then once you're at full capacity, or getting to full capacity, you can start looking beyond that.

WHERE TO FIND LEVERAGE

There are many areas where salon owners struggle in terms of generating more revenue. One that I've already talked about is through pricing and not charging enough, but there are several other areas you can explore.

Average bill

Another area to look at is the average bill among your clients.

It typically costs seven to ten times more to attract a new client than it does to sell to one that you've already got, so you have to think about what you can do to encourage your clients to spend more at each visit. One way of doing this is through up-sells, or as I like to call them up-serves, where you're selling an additional service, treatment or product to your clients who are already in the salon and who are ready to pay.

Increasing the average bill makes a big difference to your business, but in my experience too many salon owners fail to see the opportunity here. In very simple terms, if you have 100 customers in a week and each one of them spends just five pounds more with you, you'll make an extra £500 a week without having to bring in any more clients. Over the course of a year, that's an additional £26,000.

Utilisation

Something as simple as keeping very tight control of your diary and making sure that you're utilising your columns effectively. You want to avoid having too many staff and not enough clients, or having staff with big gaps in their days.

Existing customers

There are three ways to grow your business. One is to get your customers to visit more often, another is to get them to spend more money when they're there, and the final one is to get more new customers. Often businesses, not just salons, become obsessed with finding new customers but they're failing to leverage the ones they already have. Making sure you book them in for their next treatment while they're there is a key step, because it means they won't leave and forget about it.

Your existing customers will spend more money with you if you give them the opportunity. As well as offering a cut and design, offer a deluxe cut and design. As well as offering colouring, offer a deluxe colour package. Deluxe manicures, facials, you name it, you can create a deluxe version of it. This is something that a lot of salons don't do but it's one that offers so much potential. They are already in your salon and they're already happy to spend money with you. Encourage them to spend a bit more and leverage the customers you already have.

HOW TO INCREASE YOUR PROFIT MARGINS

As well as knowing your numbers and pricing for profit, there are a few other areas you can focus on to improve your margins. One thing that I've seen salon owners do is go from being scared to part with any money because they're on such a shoestring budget that they see everything as a cost rather than an investment, to suddenly spending money on all kinds of things to invest in their business. However, it's important that you maximise what you have before you invest in anything new, otherwise you could find yourself investing in the wrong areas.

It's also essential to plug any gaps, which means identifying where you are overspending. In my experience, most salons tend to overspend on wages and on stock. We all want our stylists and therapists to make as much money as they can and to be happy working for us, but this can't be to the detriment of you as the owner. You have to make sure that you can afford their wages and still make a profit from your business, otherwise what's the point?

However, when you're plugging the gaps, you have to be very careful that you don't strike off the things that are actually making you money. All too often people will view marketing or education as a cost rather than an investment, which means they can strike them off when they're plugging the gaps. You can't afford to do this. You need that knowledge and you need to invest in these areas, otherwise you're just keeping yourself stuck in your struggle.

UNDERSTANDING MARKETING COSTS

One area that it is always worth investing in is marketing. Doing this well can have a big impact on your profit margins, but it's important to understand that marketing costs you either time, money or both. Either way, it's an investment and it's one that you have to get used to because having a marketing budget is very important. You also need to look closely at the return you get on your marketing.

For example, let's say that I helped a salon create a Facebook advert on a budget of £20. I will always ask the salon how that advert performed and ask what they got back from it. I might get a response like, 'Well, it didn't really go that well, we only got two new customers from it.'

I'd then ask, 'What did those customers spend?' They might say, 'Oh, they both had colours and spent £80 each.' That means that advert, which cost the salon £20, brought in £160. The return on that is incredible. But I often find that people struggle to get their head around the return that these kinds of marketing investments can bring. I then ask, 'Would you give me £20 if I gave you £160 in return? How many £20 notes would you find if you knew you were getting £160 in return for each one?'

Even getting one new customer from an advert and breaking even is good, because you have to look at what that customer will go on to spend with your business if they come back again. Marketing shouldn't be viewed as a cost, but as an investment. However, to really appreciate that, you need to make sure you always look at the return on that investment.

If you find that an advert is working well, don't stop using it. The reasons to switch off an advert are because it's stopped working or it's not bringing in the right quality of client. There should always be a genuine reason rather than getting a few customers in, thinking it was great and then just stopping that advertising. This is all about playing the long-term game, rather than looking for instant gratification.

CHAPTER 7

RETURN

This is really all about how you can get your customers to visit your salon more often and spend more while they're with you. Remember that I talked about the three ways you can grow your business in the last chapter? You can get your customers to visit more often, you can get them to spend more while they're in the salon or you can find new customers.

The impact of leveraging each of these areas can be much greater than you might imagine. Just look at the example below:

- Average bill £35 - 476 clients visit 6 times a year (every 8 weeks) = 2856 visits
  x £35 = £99,960
  +10% to average bill = £38.50
  +10% to client amount = 523
- +2 extra visits a year
- (6 week rebook instead of 8) = 4184 visits

- **Times your average bill by # visits**
- 38.50 x 4181 = £160,968.50

Growth 61%

- **Which area gives most growth?**
- 10% increase in average bill only = £109,956
- 10% increase in client numbers alone = £109,830
- Just one visit a year more by each client = £116,620
- Two more visits per client = £133,280

What you want to look at is what would happen to your returns if you just increased each of those areas by a small increment, let's say 10%. In the example above, your salon is turning over £99,960 a year and you do nothing more than get each of your customers to spend 10% more on each visit, you'll be making an extra £9,996 in a year.

If you only increase the number of customers coming to your salon by 10% the outcome is about the same, so an additional £9,870 a year.

However, as soon as you start to add on, you see the figures jump up more quickly. For example, if each customer comes for just one more visit in a year, that will increase your revenue by around £16,600 a year. If you can get them to come for two more visits a year, that's an extra £33,200 in revenue. That means you could go from turning over £99,960 at your salon to turning over £160,000, just by leveraging the customers you already have.

What this example shows you is the importance of getting your clients to rebook. In the salon industry we all know that it's important, but once you work it out in terms of what that would mean to your business you can suddenly see the huge difference it could make.

This is what return is all about. It's the strategy you can use to make sure your customers keep coming back and that they come back more often.

Focusing on getting your existing customers to come to your salon more often, rather than focusing on getting new customers through the door, helps in a number of ways. Firstly, it means that the average bill per customer goes up. Secondly, it helps with your marketing budget because each time someone comes back to your salon, you're getting greater return on your marketing investment to bring them in initially.

Often salons focus too much on bringing new customers in to fill the empty spaces this week, rather than focusing on finding new customers for life. It's important to think long term and have a strategy to encourage your customers to increase the frequency of their visits.

HOW CAN YOU GET YOUR CUSTOMERS TO RETURN?

View your new customers like dates

Whenever you get a new client, you have to remember that you want that new client to return, and if you can get them to come back to you three times, they're yours. It's only you who can mess it up after that. One thing I often advise people to do is view their new customers like dates.

Imagine you go on a first date, and then you have a second and a third date within a week. You're going to get to know them and build a bond with them really quickly. Even if you see them once a week for three weeks, you're going to form that bond. When it comes to your customers, three times in three months is still okay, but your strategy should always be to get that new customer back to your salon three times as quickly as you possibly can. You want to build that relationship as quickly as you can.

Rather than telling a new customer you'll see them again in six weeks, or eight weeks or ten weeks, you want to get them back much sooner than that to build the relationship. I'll even give something away for free to do that and get them back into my salon as soon as possible. For example, if they've come in for a cut and I can get them back in that same week for a free blow dry with a quiet graduate stylist, I'll do that. You're also helping your customer to create a new habit of visiting the salon more often.

You can't afford to allow people to leave without rebooking and you need to give them a reason to return. You can't let them walk out of your door and then just hope for the best.

Give your new customers a welcome pack

This is one of the things that we do at my salon. We give every new customer a little welcome pack and within that is what we call our little bonus book, which is basically giving them reasons to return. It might include a voucher for our makeup services, or the offer of a free blow dry, or money off a colour, but these offers are only valid for a short period of time. This scarcity encourages the booking rather than them forgetting about the offer.

Giving money off or free services is fine, because that's part of my strategy to get each new customer to come back three times as quickly as possible. I'm building that relationship with them and creating the new habit of frequency.

If you don't want to offer discounts at your salon that's fine, but then you have to think about what strategy you're going to use to get each new customer to come back three times within three weeks. You might offer them an incentive to bring a friend, or give them a free product if they come back within a week. What you offer your new customers to get them back into your salon doesn't really matter, it just has to be something that moves them to come back quickly.

> 'I attended a Salon Jedi bootcamp on March 10th, I remember as it was my birthday. I had seen the Facebook advert and listened to Caroline's story which resonated with my own. I remember thinking what a remarkable woman, what's her secret?
>
> For the first time in many years I felt I had hope. I knew in the first hour I was hungry for more and eagerly signed up for the two-day training school.'
>
> - *Amanda Allan, Heavenly Sensations*

CHAPTER 8

RETAIN

In the previous chapter I talked about how you get your customers to come back three times in those early weeks and I said that you should treat it like dating. Retain is the next step on from that, it's about how you keep your customers for life. So, if return was like dating, retain is like marriage. There are several ways you can keep your customers coming back to you and I'll talk you through some of the most effective in this chapter.

MEMBERSHIPS

Memberships are a great way to retain clients because they tie them into your salon, as opposed to just one stylist. I launched a membership package at my salon back in 2012 and I was one of the first salons to take this approach.

When I talk about a membership I mean getting a client to buy a membership package for a year, six months or even three months in advance. If someone has bought one of those packages and their preferred stylist leaves, they're much less likely to follow them because they are tied into this package with the salon. When someone has a membership like this at my salon, generally their treatments and cuts will be done with their main stylist, but there are other services that they'll get from other members of the team. For example, the stylist doesn't do the blow dry, a graduate does that. Or if their preferred stylist was on holiday, they would be booked in with someone else at the salon.

This means that they get to know more members of my team and some of my clients are coming in weekly, so it feels like they're part of the family and they know everyone.

As a result, even if a stylist does leave, it's a lot less likely that they'll take all their regular clients with them. Losing a stylist is one of the biggest fears many salon owners have, because they are worried that if their stylist who is bringing in £1,000+ a week leaves, all of that money will go with them. This fear prevents them from confronting issues and dealing with problem members of staff. However, if you take the approach of building relationships between your customers and your whole team, you'll feel a lot more confident that your customers will stick with your salon even if their preferred stylist goes elsewhere.

LOYALTY CLUBS

Loyalty clubs are another great way to retain your customers, where you provide them with a rebooking incentive. At my salon we have a colour club, for example, and anyone who is in that club gets a loyalty card that allows them to build up points and prizes. We're giving them more reasons to come to us more often and choose us for colour, and not reach for the box.

REACHING OUT TO LOST CLIENTS

If one of the stylists at my salon leaves and some of our clients go with them, our marketing clicks in straight away. We'll give clients opportunities to try other stylists and we'll make it feel really easy and safe for them. So, we'll recommend one of our other stylists and tell them why we think they'd be a good fit. We tell them they can try this stylist and if they're not happy they can try one of our other stylists. That might mean we tell them that if they're not happy, they don't have to pay. Or it could be that we offer them a discount or a free treatment if they give our other stylist a chance.

We also send out lost-client letters to say we miss them and want them back.

It's important that if a client does leave that you give them a reason to return. Often clients who do go elsewhere can feel embarrassed to come back because they feel as though they've been disloyal to you. This is when those lost-client letters can be really effective. If they are realising that what you offered was better than what they have now, but are feeling scared or embarrassed about returning to your salon, your letter can give them a reason to return.

In our letters we might say something along the lines of, 'We miss you. We haven't seen you at the salon for a while. We'd love to see you again, so here's a shameless bribe of a Free Voucher to nudge you back. There have been a lot of changes since you were last here, etc...' Often this will encourage them to come back. The voucher will have quite a short expiry date on it, because you want to get them back in as soon as you can. If we don't get a response to our first letter, we send a second one. I can tell you that our second letter always gets a better response than the first letter.

This brings me on to another fear that people have when it comes to marketing. They worry that they are marketing too much to their customers, but I believe that you have to view this as a relationship worth fighting for. If you just let customers leave and follow the stylist that left your salon, without doing anything to try and bring them back, it's as though you don't care. I feel that it's my duty to show our clients how much we care about them, how much we value the relationship with them and how much we want them back.

In the second letter, I say something along the lines of, 'Hi, it's Caroline again. I noticed that you have not utilised the gift voucher I sent you but I've just had a thought that you might have been on holiday, or maybe you recently had your hair done, so what I've done is extended the expiry date on that voucher for you.' You might even increase the offer to give them an extra nudge to come in.

You could also consider sending a third and final letter, which we've done at my salon in the past as well. One of the things we used to offer in that final letter was for a client to come and try our new stylist for free because we were so confident they would love them. At that point the client has nothing to lose and it can be a good way to get them back through your door.

Advice on writing letters

I would recommend that any letters you send out are printed in a handwritten font so that it looks more personal. You don't have to sit and handwrite all your letters yourself. The letters from my salon all feature a picture of me and they come from me directly as the salon owner. This is important if you have stepped away from the floor, like I have, because it allows you to build that relationship with the clients as well.

Always handwrite the name and address on the envelope though. When you think about it, seeing a handwritten envelope among the printed brown and white envelopes containing bills and junk mail is quite rare. That means your letter will grab their attention straight away and make them curious.

Of course you have the option of emailing or texting your clients instead, but in this instance, although direct mail costs more to send, I've always found that it gets a better response than those other options.

> *'[Caroline] is inspirational as a businesswoman that has had the same problems as me and come out the other side smiling. Her ideas are amazing and best of all..... they work! The support network that Caroline has created is something I don't think I could be without now.'*
>
> -   **Emma Simmons, Salon 54**

BUILDING RELATIONSHIPS WITH NEW CLIENTS

Following on from this, all of the new clients at my salon receive a letter thanking them for visiting the salon and reminding them that they've got an offer to come back to the salon in the next couple of weeks. In this letter I also ask if they enjoyed their visit and then remind them that they can leave us a review if they are happy. I also say that if they're not happy for any reason, they can get in touch and I make sure that I include my email address and tell them to let me know if there's anything more that I can do.

How many hairdressing or beauty salons have you been to in your life that have sent out this kind of letter shortly after you've visited them for the first time? There are very few salons that will do this, but it's something I've done for years and have always found it to be a great way to retain clients and get them back to my salon as soon as possible after their first visit.

SEND OUT TEXT OR EMAIL REMINDERS

We send out text message and/or email reminders to our clients, reminding them that their haircut is due, and if they haven't visited us by 11 weeks then we send out a reminder saying, 'Did you realise it's been 11 weeks since your last haircut? Give us a call and let's get you booked in.' We get a lot of positive responses to that reminder.

We also use text message reminders with new clients. So, as I mentioned, we send them an offer in the new-client letter and a few days before it's due to expire we'll send them a text reminder. After that expiry date passes, we'll send them another offer for the next few weeks, which isn't as good as the first offer but still provides an incentive for them to book back in within the next six weeks.

This is all part of the client journey that I've worked out for my business. It starts with their welcome letter, then we move on to the text and email reminders and then, if they haven't booked in again within 16 weeks, they become a lost client and we go back to the letters.

USING SOCIAL MEDIA

Our Facebook strategy is an important part of the overall marketing strategy at my salon. If we come back to the dating analogy, you wouldn't just walk up to somebody you don't know in a bar and ask them to marry you. You'd want to be seen by them first and flirt a little, and then perhaps swap numbers and start dating.

We use our social media, and specifically Facebook, to be seen by potential new clients. We do that using video because it allows us to remarket really well to anyone who watches the video. Within the beauty industry, before, during and after videos are great. They work very well because they tell a complete story, starting with the pain of having bad hair and finishing with the transformation.

People watch these videos to the end because they want to see the result, and because they've watched that video, Facebook will then register that they're interested. We also use a Facebook pixel on our website, which not only allows you to track conversions from your Facebook ads, but also helps you to remarket to anyone who has interacted with your website.

There's one video for my salon that has had 156,000 views. This performed so well because I targeted it to the local community and I put some money behind it. With videos like this, I create them to target the people I want to see them, my avatar, and then once someone has watched a video, Facebook picks them up and I can then add them to a custom audience on Facebook and retarget them with adverts.

The key point with this initial video content is that you're not trying to sell anyone anything. It's just like flirting in a bar, you just want to be noticed. If you think about it like this, the next stage would be dating and if everything goes well with your flirting you'd be swapping numbers. Eventually you can sell to people, but in these initial stages it's important that you're not asking for anything, you're just showing them something that's entertaining or educational. Only once I've built the custom audience of video viewers (flirted) will I then retarget them with an advert with a call to action (ask for a date).

Social media is also an important tool for making sure that you stay front of mind for your clients. Before the likes of Facebook, when someone left your salon they wouldn't see you or hear from you in the six to eight weeks between their appointments. Now you're able to make sure that you're in front of them during that period by maintaining an active presence on social media.

WHERE YOU CAN'T AUTOMATE YOUR MARKETING, SYSTEMISE

Many of the things I've just talked about, such as sending out emails and text messages, can be automated. It's important that you leverage your time, which means taking advantage of technology where you can.

However, when it comes to sending out physical letters, this isn't a process that you can automate. It is, however, one that you can systemise. I'll talk more about systems in Part 4 of the book, but I'll explain the system we have in place for dealing with this at my salon.

Every Monday, we look at the new clients from last week and we make sure that letters go out to all of them. This is part of our system and someone on the team has that job of printing out the letters and posting them each week. You should also have a system for sending out your lost-client letters and any other direct mail campaigns you plan to run. It could be as simple as having a note in the diary every quarter for someone to check that list and send those letters out. So even though you can't fully automate this process, you can systemise it.

Facebook marketing can be a combination of the two. There are some elements of our Facebook marketing that are automated and consistently run, such as scheduling the posts designed to attract new customers, but there are other elements that we change based on whatever strategy we're working on at the time. It's very important that you have a strategy for your social media and that you're not just posting on Facebook when you're quiet. We have standby offers, like last-minute deals that we can use to fill late cancellations, but we use them sparingly.

That's because we have built a very strong list and we typically send out these kinds of offers to the people on our list rather than scrambling around on Facebook to fill gaps in our diary. For example, at my salon we have a WhatsApp group of customers, we have a customer Facebook group and we have VIP subscribers on our website who choose to receive marketing from us, and we have our salon database. What that means is that we have several very strong lists that we can send out offers to or even just updates to. The key is to always be thinking ahead and strategising. It's always better to be too busy and turning people away than not busy enough.

You have to keep your marketing going all the time. You can turn it up or turn it down, but you never switch it off.

ACKNOWLEDGEMENT

This refers to acknowledging things like anniversaries, just like you would in any relationship. The biggest reason you will lose a customer is complacency, because people want to feel like they're being listened to and they want to feel heard. If we don't feel as though we're heard and seen, that isn't a good relationship.

It's very important that you don't take your long-term customers for granted. You should acknowledge their birthdays, or anniversaries in terms of how long they've been supporting your business. You can tell them how much you appreciate them for being one of your longest-standing customers, or acknowledge their first-year anniversary. However you do it, it's just important to acknowledge them. If you don't do this and start to be complacent about them, you will lose them. It doesn't matter if they've been coming to you for 20 years, if they don't feel appreciated they will go elsewhere. Make them feel seen and listened to. You have to work on their loyalty with every visit and use every appointment as an opportunity to cement that relationship.

ALWAYS COME FROM A PLACE OF GIVING

I often encounter salon owners who are resistant to giving discounts at their business, or who are scared of giving discounts to their existing customers, but will discount for new customers coming in. My advice is to always approach any offer that you're running from a place of giving.

You should make sure that you take just as much care, if not more, with your existing customers as you do with your new customers. You should want to reward loyalty and make them feel joyful and happy.

I would also say that the key to making the most of any offers that you run is to be very clear on the terms and conditions attached. There are several reasons for this. Firstly, this is about managing expectations and making sure that your customers don't go away disappointed if they try to redeem an offer on a day it's not valid. So, if an offer isn't valid on a particular day (such as a Saturday) make sure that it's very clear to your customers.

If someone does come in with a voucher that isn't valid on Saturday, for example, but that's about to expire, I would extend it for another week or maybe two to allow them to use it. What I won't do, however, is let them use that voucher on a Saturday, because if you do this then you're essentially telling them that the terms don't matter. You need to find a way of working around it and offering a solution that you're happy with.

Sticking to your terms and conditions is very important when you're running offers. If you only have ten of something to give away, make sure that you do only give away ten. If you change your mind, you can always reopen the offer at a later date to give away another ten. You want to make sure that when you say an offer is limited that you mean it. Otherwise you'll have customers calling you asking if you have any offers on and they'll be expecting offers each time they book. You need to make your offers feel special and you don't want your customers to believe that they're ten a penny.

Remember it's not always about the offer. Yes, there are times to use these strategically, for example to get your three visits from new clients, but things like positioning yourself as the expert, shouting about awards and accreditations, using social proof like reviews, and using risk reversal (your guarantee) are all great marketing strategies.

RETAIN PROFITABILITY AS WELL AS CUSTOMERS

I've talked a lot about how to retain customers, but it's very important that you make sure you also retain profitability in your business. Whatever you do to retain your customers, you always need to ensure that you're retaining profitability at the same time.

As I mentioned in Chapter 6, if you don't put your prices up but your costs increase, you gradually become less and less profitable. Even if you're retaining your customers, they will become less and less profitable if you don't increase your prices as other expenses go up. I often encounter salon owners who are scared of increasing prices for their regulars, but it's essential to retain the profitability of each customer otherwise you are the one who will lose out.

CASE STUDY
KRYSIA WEST

I'm Krysia West and I own Perfectly Posh Hair Design. I opened my salon in November 2007 and by April 2008 a recession had been declared in the UK. It was far from an ideal time to open a new business. On a personal level, it was particularly challenging as my first marriage broke down just a month after I'd opened the salon. That meant money was really tight as I'd been relying on my husband's income to support me while I built my business.

However, the first year to 18 months the salon did really well, but then I started to notice that people weren't coming in every six weeks for their haircuts. Instead they were leaving it ten or even 12 weeks between cuts. More people were starting to dye their hair at home. Even though I was running what I'd describe as a competitive salon on price, where a cut and blow dry was £25 for instance, I began to struggle as the recession hit my potential clientele particularly hard.

I was losing more and more money because people were coming into the salon less and less often. My first husband also left me with a lot of debt and I was really struggling to get out of that financial hole. I knew I needed to do something, so I started researching how I could make more money at my salon and that's how I found Caroline. Her story spoke to me and even though her situation was different to mine, the financial challenges she faced were very similar. This was in 2009/10 and Caroline had just started Salon Jedi, so I got in touch with her to ask for help.

I joined her Salon Jedi programme and I implemented everything that she recommended. I was often working till 1am in the morning, eating my dinner at my computer after getting home from work and putting my daughter to bed. After about a year, I started to see a difference and my salon started to grow.

What was interesting was that I started seeing other salons in my area copying what I was doing, because they'd obviously noticed that my business was growing, but often it didn't work for them because they didn't understand how or why I was doing certain things. Caroline's training was a secret weapon for me. She opened my eyes up to what was out there and she opened my eyes to what marketing could achieve.

The possibilities of marketing

I was a stylist who opened a salon. I didn't have a clue about marketing and I didn't know how to run my business. I knew how to work in my business but I didn't know how to run it and that's an important difference.

Caroline's model and strategies helped me grow my business substantially. Her foundation model is all about repeating what you're doing well and that was always there for me. The marketing side of it was definitely what helped me build and grow my business, and without her guidance on marketing, I probably would have gone under because I wouldn't have known how to market myself.

Strategies that work

I've been using some of Caroline's marketing strategies for years because they work. One great example is Buy One, Get One Free vouchers. The first year I offered these, I think I made about £1,000, but each year the amount grew: £1,000 became £3,000; £3,000 became £7,000; then £15,000. The most I've made in one day with those vouchers is £25,000.

This just goes to show how effective Caroline's strategies are, and they're as relevant now as they were when I started with her back in 2009.

The key is commitment

I remember someone in the group who was working with Caroline at the same time as me sometimes saying that certain strategies weren't working and I'd always ask them if they were doing 100% of it, because if you aren't committed to these strategies, they won't work.

The marketing ties in with what Caroline teaches about your mindset. If you believe in it, it's going to happen, but if you have negativity or don't believe something will work, then it won't. I committed fully to everything she taught, and I wasn't afraid of something not working out because she had taught me that's what marketing is all about: testing and improving. That was an important element of what she taught.

Going from strength to strength

I can say with certainty that I wouldn't be where I am now, in my third salon, making the kind of money I'm making now, without Caroline to support and guide me through those early years because I wouldn't have known how to get through those challenges without her.

When I started my salon, I took out a five-year lease on the premises. When this lease came to an end I'd been working with Caroline for four years. I had grown so much in that period that I had to move to a bigger salon. Five years after making that move, I've tripled my business again. In less than a decade I've grown my business more than I would have thought possible when I first started out.

I have gone from earning £1,000 a week to sometimes earning £10,000 a week. I've gone from having one stylist to having six or seven stylists. I've gone from being the most competitive salon to the most expensive salon in my town, and I've gone from being the smallest salon to being the biggest and cemented my place as number one in my town, which is what Caroline specialises in.

Learning that lasts a lifetime

One of the things that Caroline encouraged us to do on her Salon Jedi course was get a notebook and write down our dreams. One of my dreams when I started was to earn £5,000 a week, and when I hit that, I wrote a new dream to earn £10,000 a week. I don't hit that every week, but I try to. She taught me to set the bar high and that means that I've achieved so much more.

Since working with Caroline, I've done other business courses as well and after every single one of them I always come back to what Caroline taught me. They act as a nice refresher and they're a good way to keep my knowledge up to date, but I would say that everything I do in my business now goes back to what Caroline taught me in 2009/10.

It's like riding a bike, you never forget. Sometimes you need a little reminder, and it's always good to revisit the fundamentals because it's easy to stop appreciating what you already have and what you've achieved.

DO YOU NEED MORE CLIENTS COMING TO YOUR SALON? IF YOU WOULD LIKE TO BOOK A FREE BREAKTHROUGH DISCOVERY CALL, SCAN THE QR CODE BELOW USING YOUR MOBILE PHONE'S CAMERA AND SELECT THE TIME THAT WORKS FOR YOU.

This breakthrough call is to look inside your business to see how to improve profits, scalability and leverage, and to identify any limiting beliefs holding you back.

We will help you discover what is not working in your salon business and plan how to scale up and reach your dream profits, even while getting off the tools if you wish.

PART 3

MANAGEMENT

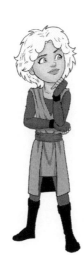

In the first two parts of the book I talked about your mindset as the salon owner and about how to attract customers to your salon. Everything you do to bring people in, from the offers to the reasons to return, needs to be managed. On top of that, you also need to manage the team. If you don't manage all of these elements then you lose control of your salon.

A key part of this is deciding who is going to be the manager. Is it going to be you, as the salon owner, or are you going to bring someone in to take the management off your hands? If you're running a full column, doing the marketing, dealing with the finance and the operations and trying to manage the salon, is that really achievable? Someone has to manage the salon, the team, the targets and the systems that you put in place. That on its own is a full-time job.

It's also about considering the management of the systems that you want in place. As the salon owner, you'll be the visionary who says how you want things to be done, but then you need to introduce a system to manage that. I'll talk more about systems in Part 4 of the book, but it's important to understand that systems have to be managed, just like any other aspect of your salon.

You need to have these things in place, otherwise your salon will end up being chaotic, and one of the best ways to do that is to have a dedicated salon manager. With someone in this role, your salon will run more smoothly and everyone in your team will know where they stand.

In this part of the book I'm going to talk to you about the three most important elements you need to manage at your salon: staff, sales and service.

CHAPTER 9

STAFF

MY STORY

If you remember back to the first part of the book, I told you about when I thought my business was falling apart just as I was about to go on maternity leave. When I returned from my maternity leave, I only went back on the salon floor one day a week. Although I was managing the salon as well, I wasn't there every day because I had to be at home with the baby.

I became a virtual manager. Before I went on maternity leave, I introduced systems and did my best to make it as easy as possible for my team to do their job. When I returned, I introduced more systems and made sure that they were followed. I only had a small team at the salon and I wanted it to be very clear who was responsible for what. I ran a tight ship, but because of all the systems I'd introduced I was able to do that virtually.

We had formal meetings digitally and I could see the diary, which meant I could always see if something hadn't been booked in correctly. Because I'd set up so much communication with my clients and because all the letters I sent out had my email address on them, anyone who came to my salon could really easily get in touch with me if they had any questions or something wasn't quite right. Part of the work I did on the marketing was to encourage people to leave reviews in my follow-up emails, messages or letters. I would also receive all the client feedback, so I knew if someone wasn't happy or if the phones weren't being answered. It really helped me to manage the business.

All of this meant that I felt as though I had eyes at the salon even though I was only really in the salon one day a week. For a while, I even introduced a team leader of the week, where one person on my team would have responsibility for overseeing everything; because we weren't as busy at the salon then as we are now, and because I only had a small team, that worked very well.

What changed everything for me was realising that we needed more front of house help. At this point we didn't even have a front of house, let alone a manager for it. While my virtual management method had worked well to keep everything ticking over, when it came to growing it wasn't enough. I realised I needed someone there to drive the business forward, and my search for a manager began.

I could have advertised for a receptionist to answer the phones and help manage the systems front of house, like the offers and loyalty rewards we were starting to run, but I decided that wasn't what I needed. What I advertised for was a client manager with no hairdressing experience needed.

It took me a while to find the right person for the job, but one day someone applied who was phenomenal. At that point, I decided I was prepared to pay more even if that meant she would have to work fewer hours to stay within my budget for the position. When my client manager started at my salon, she was just there two days a week.

My client manager is there for the clients, hence the job title. Her job is to make sure that all the systems are being properly implemented and that the client journey is perfect. She is my eyes and my ears at the salon.

When the client manager started, she liaised between the team and the clients. She made sure the team were doing what they should be doing, like offering up service, treatments, retail and so on. She made sure the clients were rebooking every visit, and very quickly she started to work more hours. She was phenomenal, but about a year after she started working for me, she left to pursue her original career. I remember the day she sent the text message and at first being devastated as we had just opened salon number two, but I immediately shifted my mindset and decided it must be for the best and that someone better was on the way.

That was when Carla came on board. Again, she's not a hairdresser and I could tell from the start that she'd be a good fit. She is savvy, has sales knowledge and has no fear of managing the team. She's been my client manager since 2012 and, again, she started part-time and very quickly built up her hours to full-time. She drives our targets, she looks at the team's targets, upgrades them and makes sure that customers are getting everything they need. Since taking on a client manager, I've never looked back and the business has grown and grown.

What I realised very quickly after hiring a client manager was that it's a position that someone needs to be in full time. As a salon owner who's running a full column, it's not possible to do everything you need to in this role as well. I often meet salon owners who see having a front of house manager as a cost, which means they're scared of hiring someone who isn't a hairdresser, but having someone who can focus on this side of the business will help you grow, and help you grow quickly.

GETTING THE RIGHT MANAGEMENT STRUCTURE IN PLACE

As we got busier and busier, I realised we needed to bring in someone else to support Carla. She is the client manager, and is actually the managing director of the business now, and she oversees all the operations. We also have a floor manager, who is responsible for overseeing the standards of the hairdressing. They are also running a column, so it's a very different role to the client manager position.

HIRE PEOPLE BASED ON THEIR VALUES

Discovering this was a light-bulb moment for me. As stated earlier, at my salon, we don't hire people based on skills. We hire people who are aligned with our core values. Of course skills are important, but we expect anyone applying for a job to have certain skills.

I'm sure any salon owner who employs staff can relate to feeling the pressure of needing a new stylist. All of a sudden, one comes along. They have great skills and they're a brilliant hairdresser, but somewhere deep down inside you there's a niggle of a doubt. However, you're desperate for staff so you take them on, even though you know they're not quite aligned with you. This comes back to what I talked about in the mindset section, where you're choosing short-term gain and you're getting long-term pain. You might have a stylist with great skills, but if they poison the team and cause problems, sometimes this can cause you issues for years.

It's not that they're bad people, just that they have different values to you and it's a mismatch. For example, imagine you're specifically looking for someone with a brilliant work ethic who will go the extra mile and who's not only passionate about hairdressing but also passionate about doing a good job on a personal level. They have that drive to do a good job and they're a team player. If that's what you're looking for and you attract someone who is a brilliant hairdresser, but who is focused on doing less for more, they're not going to be a good fit. They'll be intent on getting out of the door as fast as they can at the end of each day. They won't stay to help the rest of the team clean up. That's because their highest value is getting home to their partner or kids, or going out, or whatever it might be. It's not that those things are wrong, but if those are higher up their list of values than working as part of the team and always going the extra mile, they aren't going to fit in with your salon and the rest of your staff.

All that happens is that both parties end up being unhappy. They're unhappy because you're asking them to stay behind and do this work that they don't value. You're unhappy because you feel as though they aren't doing their job properly. It's a disaster.

You should also remember that people's values can change. It might be that someone who's always put the salon first and gone the extra mile has a baby, and then their family becomes their highest value while their work and career fall way down their values list, so their behaviour changes. That's understandable and it's not about one of you being right or wrong, it's just a case of recognising that your values aren't aligned any more. More often than not, when this happens these members of staff tend to just drift away.

The key thing as a salon owner is to understand this and understand that it's not your fault that a person's behaviour has changed.

One of the most important things you should take from this chapter is that there's nothing wrong with hiring based on your values, and you should not change your values to fit a team member. This really changed things for me and now it's part of the interview and hiring process. We don't just have one interview with new members of staff, we have several. We also have trial periods and make our values part of the induction to ensure that everyone we take on is a good fit.

HOW TO MAKE SURE YOU ATTRACT STAFF WITH THE RIGHT VALUES

The first thing to focus on is the job advert itself. Make sure you're clear and specific about the values you're looking for in your employees. When we're writing a job advert, we'll often include something along the lines of: 'This job is for you if you value self-development and want to improve your skills, value customer care and value climbing the career ladder.'

We'll often also include some text telling people what we're not looking for. It might be something along the lines of: 'This job is not for you if you want to sit in the staffroom and drink coffee when you don't have a client in.' This is to repel the stylist or therapist who is not aligned with your values.

When it comes to the interview, we're always trying to find out about their highest values. We listen very carefully to what each person says in their interview, and sometimes we can tell just by the words they're using and the way in which they're speaking what it is that they value. Another thing we do during interviews is give each person a values list and ask them to put it in order, like the one you completed earlier in the book.

We also want to see if they've done any research on the company and whether they know anything about us, or whether they're just looking for any job. We make sure we're very clear at the interview stage who we are, what our values and standards are, and what we are and aren't looking for in our team members. We also explain why it benefits both of us to make sure we're aligned in our values.

We hire slow and fire fast. It's not just a case of having one interview and then that's it. Normally we'll start with an initial chat over the phone or in the salon. Carla, my manager, usually does this. It's a disqualification process for us and she'll only pass on people for me to interview who are genuine potential candidates. This is never about the amount of CVs you receive, it's about the quality of the applicants you attract.

EDUCATE YOUR STAFF ABOUT YOUR CORE VALUES

Education is a very important part of spreading and encouraging those core values. You have to create a culture within the salon where you and your team live and breathe your core values. With younger members of staff in particular, you want to open their minds to concepts they might not have been exposed to before. Mindfulness and fostering that among your whole team is really important to help them embrace those core values, regardless of what stage they're at in their lives.

HELPING PEOPLE FLOURISH WITHIN YOUR CULTURE

Development is one of our core values, so we have a specific career ladder to help people to see the journey ahead for them. We believe it's important to help them develop and to clearly show them what they can do to work towards the next level on their career ladder. We listen to each member of staff and we make sure that we give opportunities to everyone.

For example, we have an artistic team at the salon and we give everyone an opportunity to be part of that. Often in salons, it would only be the senior members of the team who would get to be part of these kinds of activities. It costs a lot of money to do these photographic shoots, where we fly down to London and so on, but we always open this up to everyone. We might have a 16 or 17 year old going as part of the team. Now, they're not going to be doing hair and their name won't be on the finished look, but they can assist, learn and be part of the process. They have their part to play and that's an incredible opportunity.

As a salon, we enter awards and we also support our stylists to enter awards. For example, we took on a young graduate stylist when she graduated from college and within three and a half years she won Scottish hairdresser of the year, which is the biggest accolade you can possibly get in the hairdressing industry in the UK.

Our artistic team became only the second ever from a Scottish salon to be selected as finalists for the Artistic Team of the Year Award at the British Hairdressing Awards, which is a huge achievement.

All of our award entries are paid for through the company and we give our team a chance to attend the award ceremonies too. To raise the money to go to the awards in London, we would host a 'Sunday funday' where the whole team works together to raise half the money we need for the company to pay for the trip.

> *'I have had great inspiration and learning by working with Caroline for the past nine years. By focusing on growth mindset, it has helped me become one of the busiest stylists within the salon which I am extremely grateful for. She knows how to bring the best out of her team by inspiring and mentoring them.'*
>
> **-   Louise Cameron, Ego Hair Design**

HELPING PEOPLE CLIMB THE CAREER LADDER

Everyone who joins our team has clear stages of training and learning that we want them to work through. They have to reach certain levels and KPIs and so on. We have regular one-to-one meetings with each person on the team so that they know exactly where they are now and exactly what they need to do to get up to the next level.

We work hard to nurture and support every person at our salon and I would urge you to do the same. Listen to your staff, learn what their ambitions are and set out clear plans to help them achieve those while also working for the benefit of the business.

YOU HAVE TO KNOW WHO YOU ARE FIRST

Before you can start building a team, you have to be very clear on your vision and your core values. Remember that it all starts with you, so you need to know who you are and what you're doing before you start bringing other people into your team.

Once you have clarity about who you are, what you believe in and what your core values are, you'll be able to look for people who are aligned with that mission and you'll know that it's nothing personal if someone doesn't work out. It helps you to remove your emotions from situations where staff members leave and, when you have that clarity over your vision, you can see when someone isn't aligned and accept that it hasn't worked out.

MINDFUL MANAGEMENT

If you take it personally when a member of your team leaves, or when certain hires don't work out, it can set you and your salon on a downward spiral. You have to practise mindful management, which means you're not only mindful of your values, but you're mindful of other people's. You're aware of the values your team hold, but you're also aware that these can change. You do have to be mindful of that and accept that when someone isn't the right fit for your business, it's best to let them go. If they hold different values to you they'll be very difficult to manage. You could give them the world but they still wouldn't appreciate it and would still find fault with it, simply because they're not aligned with you.

You have to be strong and certain about who you are and what you stand for, but you should always be prepared to listen and tweak things if they can help you improve. What you shouldn't do, however, is make changes to align your business to someone else's values.

Although I've talked a lot about recruiting and training, there are other elements that are important when it comes to your staff and how you manage them. Our system includes a series of steps:

- Recruit (the right way).
- Rear (as in training).
- Relate (information to them).
- Review (constantly review and correct performance).
- Recognise (acknowledge results).
- Reward (when it's due).
- Raise (help them climb the career ladder).
- Reprimand (when needed).

The reason I focused so much on recruitment is because that is the most important step on that list. If you don't recruit the right person, you can forget all of the other steps because it's going to be a difficult journey.

CHAPTER 10

SALES
BY GUEST AUTHOR CARLA ZEBROWSKI

My name is Carla Zebrowski and I'm Caroline's salon manager. I've worked with Caroline for eight years and have seen the salon and academy grow by almost half a million pounds. I also work with academy clients helping them to understand their numbers and improve their sales.

As Caroline mentioned in Part 2, there are three main ways to grow your business: getting people to spend more, getting people to visit your business more often and attracting more clients. In this chapter, I share what each of those strategies looks like in practice, and share some industry secrets that can be implemented instantly and will enable you to quickly improve your sales results.

WHAT DO WE MEAN BY SALES?

To me, sales is all about giving more value to the client. It's about offering them a solution to any problem that they have. If you think about sales in general, the reason you buy something is to fix the problem of something that you need, whether it's a car, a house or a new shampoo.

WHY IS SELLING A STUMBLING BLOCK IN MANY SALONS?

The problem is that many people go through all of their hair training and then they develop this fear of selling because they think it's cold. In some stylists, this can become so ingrained that they avoid what they consider to be hard selling. However, for salon owners this is often frustrating, because they feel that the stylists should automatically be selling packages and offering products and up-serves. This all comes back to the mindset. For a stylist, it's about being mindful of what struggles the client is having and how you, as the stylist, can provide them with a solution.

What often happens is that salon owners tell their stylists that they want them to sell a particular shampoo, for instance, and the stylist doesn't understand why. They just feel like they're being forced to sell that shampoo for the sake of it. There's a disconnect between the owner and their stylists, and there is a limiting belief surrounding sales for many stylists that makes them feel uncomfortable or fearful of selling to clients.

As the salon owner, what you have to do is work on their mindset. You have to introduce them to the perspective that they're serving not selling. It's about showing them that what they're offering will help their customers, rather than allowing them to continue to hold this limiting belief about selling and to be fearful of making sales.

You have to understand where this fear has come from and work on the root cause of it. This is about far more than simply teaching someone to sell. You have to help your stylists understand what you're actually offering and show them how these products or services are solutions for your clients' problems. Once they are able to approach sales from the point of view of satisfying clients and helping them, that fear disappears.

CARLA'S STORY

I've been working with Caroline at Ego Hair Design since June 2012, when I joined as Client Manager to take care of the front of house at the salon, but my background isn't in hairdressing or even the beauty industry. Before working with Caroline, I had run my own hotel, I'd worked in a bank, been a visual merchandiser for a global company and I'd worked for Virgin. That meant I had some sales experience from my time in those retail roles, as well as from party planning and aspects of hospitality.

What I was missing was the full mindset, which is something that Caroline helped me work on. Working on my mindset was one of the first things Caroline did when I started and I think that's what made the big difference.

She explained her mindset and introduced me to books on mindfulness and meditation, which obviously help with your mindset. This knowledge, combined with the fact that I approached selling from the point of view that it is how to deliver exceptional customer service rather than a way of getting more money in the till, meant that I took to it quite naturally.

As I've already mentioned, it's about serving not selling. The aim is always to find solutions to your client's problems and very much focusing on that client journey.

Working on my own mindset is only part of this job. I also have to introduce this mindset to the rest of the team and we carry out ongoing training with them to help them view sales as a way of delivering exceptional customer service. This isn't something that happens overnight; it's an ongoing process and you have to help people who are nervous or fearful about selling to customers overcome that and see the process from a different point of view. I lead from the front and encourage them to do the same.

FOCUS ON THE TEAM

As I mentioned, encouraging the right mindset around sales within the team is a very important part of my job. This is a process that takes time and no one is going to change their approach overnight, so it has to be a team effort. I take the time to work with any team members who are a bit unsure about the approach. I'll make suggestions of services or products that could benefit a client and I'll work with them to offer those services and help them see that the client is happier as a result. It's all about showing your team members that the client benefits from this and giving them the confidence to offer extra services or products to different clients. I even buddy up with them for support and help close their sales.

AUTHENTICALLY LED SALES

To help people get into the right mindset for selling, we ask them to ask clients the specific question, 'What is important to you about your hair/skin/hairstyle?' This drives authentically led sales, because by finding out what's important to the customer you can recommend something that will be of benefit and add value to them.

For example, if you ask a customer, 'What's important to you about your hairstyle?' and their response is, 'It's got to have shine', the stylist can then consultatively sell to them. In that example they might be able to say, 'Ok, we have this product and it will give your hair a great shine.'

This is a really effective tactic to use with stylists who have that fear of selling. As soon as you get them to start asking customers this question, they're not selling any more. They're just offering solutions to a customer's problems, which makes them feel a lot more comfortable about recommending other products or services. This is the key to getting that mindset right. It's about ethical selling, because you're matching a solution to a problem. What you're advising comes with a benefit to the customer. It comes back to this idea that you're serving the customer, not selling to them.

THE ABC SYSTEM

Training this mindset of providing client benefits is the most important part of the sales training we provide to our team, but we have also created the ABC system for sales that focuses on the three main ways you can grow your business:

A – Average bill
B – Bookings
C – Clients

A = AVERAGE BILL

Increasing your customers' average bill is the first one, and there are many ways in which you can do this through marketing and through different packages that you can create at your salon. Fundamentally what we mean by average bill is that you're providing the client with more value for money. For example, you can offer up-serves, where the client pays a little more for their cut and colour, for instance, but although they pay a little extra, what they get in return is worth much more. It's all about adding value for the client, while bringing in a bit of extra money to the salon. The incredible thing about increasing the average bill is that it only needs to go up by a few pounds for each client in order for you to see a big difference in your takings each year.

Stylist/Therapist Average Bill Increase

35 clients x £40 = £1,400
38 clients x £44 = £1,672
= £272 more per week

That is just 3 clients more per week and £4 more per client
OR get 10 Clients to spend £27 more
OR get 15 Clients to spend £18 more
OR get 2 Clients to spend £136 more

Salon Average Bill Increase

100 Clients spend £40 = £4000
100 Clients spend £44 = £4400
= £400 more per week

400 x 52 weeks = £20,800 EXTRA SALES

This really is a win-win situation. Your clients get an improved service and get better value for money. Your staff earn more commission. You earn more money for the salon. Everyone is happy.

WAYS TO INCREASE YOUR AVERAGE BILL

The following are a few simple examples of ways in which you can increase your average bills.

POLO (Priority One-time Limited Offer)

This means you offer something that is only available on that day. It's a good one to do in-salon and I'd recommend running it on your busiest day of the week, such as on a Saturday. Because it's only available that day, there's a lot of urgency around it and you only make it available to the people who have come into the salon on that day.

As an example, we've run an offer where we send each client who is booked in on that day a text message in the morning telling them that if they buy a £20 voucher, they receive £10 free. In the text message, we explain that they can only get this offer if they buy the voucher today. When they arrive at the salon, we ask whether they received the text message and ask if they'd like to take us up on that offer. We find that vouchers work particularly well for these kinds of offers, because as well as encouraging them to buy the voucher, you know that they'll come back to your salon to use it.

You can also do something similar on up-serves at the salon, where you offer three for two on certain products, or you could do an offer where if someone buys a particular product, they receive a £50 voucher to spend. Those are just a few examples. The key with POLO is that it's an offer that is only available on that day.

Product packages

Like all salons, we're able to buy products in bulk. That means we can get them at a reduced price compared to retail. I'll package products up together and offer these packages to clients at an affordable price. The key to selling these packages is in how you market them.

For example, we have a leave-in conditioner that we sell, which clients can take home to help keep their hair in good condition. It's particularly useful if you have your hair coloured. A bottle will usually last around four months, so I created a package where you could buy three bottles and I marketed it as 'Have a year of haircare for XX price'. These packages flew off the salon floor.

A top tip when it comes to packages is to include a voucher in them. This not only adds more value to the client, but it encourages them to come back into the salon. It might be a voucher for a free blow dry with one of the assistants, it could be £10 off a makeup service, whatever you would like. But the key is getting them to come back into the salon.

Hair packages

The thinking behind hair packages is the same as the thinking behind product packages in that you need to offer the clients value for money. By getting your clients to come back to your salon more often, you're also building a stronger relationship with them, which is another big advantage to offering hair packages. So, when you're creating a hair package you're focusing on two things: how to give the client value for money and how to get them back in the salon.

Hair packages can offer a lot of benefits to your salon. As I've said, they allow you to build stronger relationships, but you'll also have much better client retention if you can get more of your clients to sign up to packages. You'll see an increase in bookings as well, because the nature of a package is that you'll have your regular clients coming back to the salon more frequently.

Whenever you're creating packages, there should be very clear terms and conditions. Your packages don't have to be with your top stylists, you can be very specific about who they are valid with. As the salon owner, you're in charge of who the package is with and what the timescale will be. Packages can include as much as you want them to. You can have simple cut and colour packages, for example, or you can go all the way through to memberships. Each package has to suit the business and suit the client. This isn't a case of offering huge discounts or giving everything away for free. This is about adding value to your client experiences. To do that in a way that benefits the business and the client, you need to have a strategy behind each of your packages.

The aim of packages is to get your clients to commit to coming to your salon more frequently and to pay in advance for the services they're buying. To give you an idea of how this can work, we run what we call a Superwoman package, which includes two colours and three cuts, but they have to use those within 12 to 14 weeks. The idea with this package is that when they come in for their second colour and final cut of the package, they buy the same package again for the next 12 weeks. It becomes an ongoing purchase for the customer. In buying this package, we provide a small discount on the cost of the cuts and the colours, but that's worth it, because without this package they probably wouldn't come back in as frequently. The strategy behind this package was to get our customers to come into the salon more frequently within a 12-week period and, in doing so, encourage them to spend more.

'Caroline teaches many strategies to help you build your business, but the first one we tried was a Conditioning Treatment bundle and we followed the Salon Jedi way to the letter (as much as I could, we had only just begun!) and in one email we sold 28 packages @£67 each, making £1,876. THIS WAS MY LIGHT-BULB MOMENT! Bearing in mind, in a year we had sold two conditioning treatments, this was ZERO to 28 in one email.'

- **Darren Mitzi, Darren Michael Hairdressing**

B = BOOKINGS

This still obviously relates to sales in that you're encouraging your clients to rebook sooner or getting them to book in for other services you provide. Bookings is very closely linked to the average bill, because it might be that you're able to up-serve clients to a package that includes a certain amount of services. So, instead of just coming in for their cut and colour, they're now coming in for other treatments too. That means they might come in once every seven weeks instead of once every ten, for instance. Obviously if your clients are coming in more frequently, they're spending more money with you and you're building your relationship with them. It's very important that you always show them how they're getting value for money by doing so though.

As with increasing the average bill, there are a number of ways in which you can do that. We have a three-part strategy for bookings, which is intent, instruct, incentivise.

Intent is about putting a plan in place for each client, so you have a consultation with them, you talk to them about what they want, and you decide what you're going to do with their hair and get them excited about it.

Instruct is about getting the client excited about the process. You want your clients to be excited about their next appointment so you talk them through what's going to happen over the coming weeks. If your clients know what's planned for their future appointments they're more likely to stick to them. For the stylists and the salon, this is about getting the clients to make a commitment to coming back in. The biggest mistake salons make when it comes to rebooking is asking clients, 'Would you like to rebook?' There's no urgency there. You can't assume that people will just rebook in six weeks or 12 weeks without prompting. You have to instruct them when you'd like to see them again, for example, 'I'll get you booked in for six weeks' time.' You treat it as a matter of fact that they'll be coming back. It's a bit like when you go to the dentist and they tell you that they want to see you again in six months and you just book in, often without even looking at your diary. You want people to behave the same way with their hair appointments.

Incentivise is all about giving them little rewards for rebooking, such as by running a raffle or offering a rewards card, which I'll explain in more detail below. The idea is that you're giving them an incentive to confirm that booking date before they walk out of the salon.

WAYS TO ENCOURAGE REBOOKING

Rebooking raffle

Our rebooking raffle is a good option to try. All that means is that we tell our clients that if they rebook for their next appointment before they leave the salon, they get entered into a prize draw to win a fabulous hamper or something similar. You can create a hamper using what you already have in the salon, for example end-of-line retail, wine and chocolates. Also approach local companies and ask for prizes, you will be surprised what companies will give you. Plus, remember to add a voucher to keep them returning to the salon.

Rewards card

We have a rewards card, which is particularly good for people with short hair, who tend to come in more often. For example, you might offer a reward card for anyone who books in with you every six weeks and you provide them with a reward on their third, fifth and sixth visits. You can decide what that reward should be, based on what you feel will work at your salon.

When you're incentivising rebooking, it's all about the time frame. You don't want to reward someone for booking in with you in six months' time. You want to reward them for regular and frequent rebooking.

Personal incentives

It's always worth pointing out to clients that if they block rebook then they will be guaranteed to get the appointment times that they want. If they typically want to come at busy times, such as on a late night, this is a really big draw. If they don't book in advance, there's no chance that they'll get the time slot they want every few weeks.

Focusing on booking creates another win-win situation. You have more money coming in, but the clients love the service they're receiving and they'll probably be recommending you to other people as well. It all ties back in with what we talked about in the return chapter in Part 2.

C = CLIENTS

Clients means that you're attracting more people to your salon. Obviously, if you have more clients you're going to be taking more money and your business will grow. Again, there are some very simple things you can do to attract new people to your salon.

We also have a three-step process for attracting new clients: *reach, response, referral.*

Reach means reaching out to get new clients. There are many ways of doing this and I'll share some of them further on in this chapter. Some that might come to mind can include flyering and using social media. Although a lot of people focus on digital media, it's important not to forget about marketing offline in your local community, because that's where your customers are and where they live. We've found it particularly effective to reach out to local businesses to reach more people in our area.

Response is about how you respond to the clients who are contacting you and reaching out to you. We use the rule of three, so always try to answer the phone within three rings and respond to emails or digital enquiries within three minutes. This is particularly important on social media, because if someone has sent a message on Facebook for example, they might be waiting for you to respond straight away and they might have sent a message to a few other salons, so it will be the first one to get back to them who gets the booking. It's all about having that urgency of responding when they come to you. As well as responding quickly, it's important that you respond professionally.

If you're worried that you can't physically respond quickly, or you find that responding to customer enquiries gets pushed down your list of priorities, there are systems out there that can help and that can automate some of those responses. For example, we use a call management service that sends an automated text message to any client we miss a call from telling them that we'll call them back within five minutes.

WHY IT'S IMPORTANT TO RESPOND QUICKLY

To show you why it's important to respond quickly, imagine that you're missing just one call a day and each of those calls is from a client who wants to book a £35 cut at your salon. If you're open five days a week, that means you're losing £175 a week, which equates to £9,100 a year. But it's not just the one cut that you're missing, it's the lifetime value of a new customer that you're losing out on. I'd recommend taking the time to do that very simple exercise with your salon's prices and work out how much more you could make if you were able to pick up even one more phone call a day.

Referral is the final part of the process for attracting new clients. Referrals are the easiest way to get new clients and if your clients are coming to you all the time and they love you, then they are the best people to refer you. Give them an incentive to refer you and make sure you're not just rewarding the new customer they bring in.

WAYS OF ATTRACTING NEW CLIENTS

Workplace of the Week campaign

We run a Workplace of the Week campaign, which we market and advertise in our local area and on social media. We run this campaign for a week, which gets people talking about the campaign and the salon, tagging their workplace and mates in the posts and so on. On the following Monday, we'll choose a winner at random and present them with £200 worth of vouchers. These vouchers can be split up to suit your business, so it might be that we give 20 vouchers for £10 off makeup or colour, or we offer vouchers for half-price cuts. We can be flexible about that to suit the winning business. We use this campaign if we're having a quiet period, or if we need to build up a new stylist, for example. The key is to make sure there are strict terms and conditions attached to these vouchers. Usually those vouchers have to be used within a week and they have to be used with the stylist you've specified. There is always a system behind it.

Recommend a friend incentives

If you're running this kind of system, it's very important that the person who is referring someone receives the same value as the person who is being referred. It's no good giving your new customer loads of money off their first visit and then giving nothing back to the person who referred them, because that doesn't give them any incentive to make referrals. We give referral cards to our clients and they can pass these on to their friends so that we know they've come from a referral. It's important to never give just one referral card as that implies they have just one friend. Following the rule of three, give three to nine cards. Research has shown nine to be the optimum amount to give.

You can be clever in how you market these kinds of referral schemes too. For example, if your incentive for a referral is a £10 discount on their next cut, and a cut at your salon costs £40, you could market your referral scheme as, 'Refer four friends to us and get your next cut for free!' Your existing client could then end up having a free cut, but they've brought you four new clients who each get £10 off their first cut with you too. It's all about framing your referral incentives to show your clients what's in it for them.

Referral clubs

When Ego Hair Design moved to a bigger salon in 2012 it was to accommodate 2,000 new clients, and the biggest source of those clients was referrals. We had a referrals club called our Ego Maniacs Club and it proved really popular. Firstly, our marketing said 'Join our referrals club and get up to £200 of free hairdressing and treatments'. That was enough to get people to ask about it. When they did, we'd sign them up and give them nine referral cards. The deal we were offering was that the client would get a £15 discount and a free treatment for every person they referred. The friends they referred would get the same on their first visit. If they used all nine of those cards, they could get up to £200 worth of discounts and treatments. The key was making it feel like a club and very clearly showing them not only what was in it for them, but also what was in it for their friends.

Reward cards

If you offer reward cards to your clients, either for referring someone or regularly booking appointments, it's important to remember that you can change the rewards you're giving out to suit your business. You might offer a discount with a particular stylist if their diary is a bit quiet. Or you might provide products if you're really busy with bookings.

TRAINING YOUR TEAM IS KEY

Whatever offers you're running, it's important that you always put these in front of your customers. Your marketing is one way of doing that, which we discussed extensively in Part 2, but your staff and front of house are also essential to this.

As I've already said, once you train your staff to think differently about sales, they'll feel less nervous about making recommendations to their customers. It's important that you also make sure they know about the latest offers you're running, so you have to educate your team as well as keeping your marketing up to date.

We also make it as easy as possible for our team to make our clients feel special. Each stylist has their own cards that they have at their station or in their pouch. These cards have discount vouchers or are referral cards and they can personally give them to their clients. This adds a personal touch to it and makes our clients feel very special and feel as though their stylist values them.

It's important to understand that this is an ongoing process. It's not a case of you teaching your team once and then all of a sudden they're phenomenal sales people. This is a process that you have to maintain and monitor.

OFFER ALTERNATIVES RATHER THAN SAYING 'NO'

On occasion people will come in with an expired voucher, or maybe they didn't use the final couple of blow drys that were part of a package they bought a year ago and they want to use one of them now. You have to be very careful how you manage these customers. Obviously your terms and conditions are important, but if you just say 'No' and turn them away, then you're not giving them a good experience and chances are that you'll lose them.

Depending on what it is, I will normally explain that their voucher has expired but then I'll offer them an alternative. It might be a discount voucher that they can use another time, it might be that I'll tell them they can book in for a free blow dry if they come next week. You have to read the situation but the key is to give them something so that they still feel like they're getting value rather than missing out, and which still suits the business needs and availability.

THE IMPORTANCE OF FRONT OF HOUSE

Front of house plays an essential role in the sales at your salon and not just the sales of the products, but also the sales of hair services. Your front of house staff should be up-serving customers, making them aware of any packages or offers that are available to them and so on.

Front of house is also vital in terms of picking up the phone and converting those enquiries into bookings or consultations. As I mentioned earlier, the cost of not replying to enquiries quickly can be huge.

As a front of house manager, it's also my job to maintain and monitor the sales training I talked about earlier among the team. I have to make sure that I'm regularly updating everyone's training and educating them. I've got to keep an eye on each team member's mindset to make sure that they don't slip back into their old way of thinking, where they become fearful of selling again.

It's also important that I check that every member of the team is still carrying out the consultations correctly and asking all the right questions of their clients to make sure that each person is getting value for money.

One thing we introduced was a consultation card, which worked really well. When a client came in for a consultation, I'd give them a consultation card to fill in before they went to their stylist. It was a very simple checklist that asked questions about their hair type and what information they'd be interested in hearing during their consultation. So, we asked questions about whether they wanted to know more about different products or home haircare and so on. Once they'd filled it in, they just handed it to their stylist at the beginning of the consultation. That meant they had all this information about the client and what they were interested in, which broke the ice and gave the stylists confidence to talk about other products or services that would benefit that client.

Although there was an option on this card to say that they didn't want any information, no one ever ticked that box. This is just a simple example of a system you can put in place at front of house that makes the sales process easier and smoother for both your team and your clients.

If you've got a team in your salon and are struggling to grow your sales, you can view the full consultation checklist we give to our clients at the end of the chapter.

It's important to understand that a front of house role is about more than answering phones and greeting clients. Your staff in this area have a vital role to play in growing your business and they're integral to the sales process.

Name:
Prescription:

CONSULTATION CARD

Ego Hair Design
five star hair care

To help us give you everything you need at your visit, please answer the following questions:

Tick the 3 things most important to you about your hair:

Volume ☐	Shine ☐	Condition ☐
Smooth ☐	Moisture ☐	Always looking its best ☐
Clean Blonde ☐	Fresh Colour ☐	On Trend ☐
Other ☐		

What are the 3 most important things you would like to receive from your stylist today, alongside a great service?

Getting home care advice ☐	Getting advice on improving condition ☐
Receiving value for month ☐	Advice on salon savings ☐
Relaxing back wash service ☐	No advice ☐
Other ☐	

At future visits, which is the most important to you?

Having the best, most experienced stylists ☐   Having the cheapest stylists ☐

Please tick here if you would **NOT** like to receive any advice or offers from your stylist today ☐

CHAPTER 11

SERVICE

We use service as an acronym, with each of the elements making up what I consider to be a super salon service!

S – Standards
E – Educate
R – Relate
V – Value
I – Inform
C – Care
E – Elevate

STANDARDS

This obviously refers to our standards, but it's important to remember that we'll get more of what we tolerate. This is really important when it comes to your service and who you are as a brand, because if you drop your standards anywhere and that lower standard is allowed to continue, it has a knock-on effect. That means if one member of your team lowers their standards and you allow that to happen, the rest of the team will see that and it will become a new, lower standard.

From there, standards will continue to fall. As the salon manager, you have to step in as soon as you see standards dropping to make sure that they never start to slide. This is about managing the standards of service to make sure that they stay high.

When you're busy or you're stressed or you just want to avoid confrontation, it can be very easy to see that your standard isn't being met but then you get distracted, you forget, or you avoid doing anything about it. However, as I said at the start of this section, you'll get more of what you tolerate and this is how standards begin to slide. It comes back to what I talked about in Part 1, where you have to accept some short-term pain for that long-term gain. In the short term it might be painful to address the behaviour you've seen and fix it if it doesn't meet your standards, but in the long term this will pay off.

EDUCATE

It goes without saying that you should always be educating your team, but in the context of service we're talking about educating your clients. That might mean educating them about how they can do their hair at home, such as by giving them some quick tips on how to style their hair in different ways or telling them about a home hair care regime or, for beauty salons, home skin care regimes. It might also be that while you're chatting to them, you explain why you're cutting their hair in a certain way, or why you're using a particular product.

All the chatter that you have with them doesn't just have to be about holidays and what you did at the weekend, you can use that time to educate your clients and add more value to their experience. Clients really appreciate this and it helps you build a stronger relationship with them.

The other way to think about education is that if you were to buy an expensive shirt, it would have a care label in it that tells you how to wash it and how to look after it. Imagine that you're doing a colour on someone's hair and you make it look lovely when they walk out of the salon door, but if you haven't educated them about how they can look after their colour and maintain their hair at home, that expensive colour that you've done for them could go down the drain. This could be the same for beauty treatments.

Education also includes managing expectations. Tell them what they can expect when they first wash their hair and how they can style it the way you have. Educate them about what comes next, such as how often they need to come back for a cut or a colour. If you're giving them a goody bag that includes vouchers, educate them about what's in it. Tell them about the products, but also point out that the vouchers expire, so you're encouraging them to use them sooner rather than later.

RELATE

When it comes to service, I'm talking about relating to your customers and being able to communicate with them in a way that suits them. For example, if you've got a client who's very quiet, timid and softly spoken, it's about respecting how they're presenting and coming onto their level. That might mean you take your energy levels down a notch and speak more quietly.

Relate also means being able to relate to your client's emotional state, so recognising if they seem a bit sad or happy and communicating with them in a way that shows that you're aware and mindful of how they're feeling.

This doesn't just apply to clients who are in the salon; it's the same on the phone. If, like me, you tend to talk quickly, you might need to slow down a little for some people if they're more measured in how they talk.

Being able to relate to your clients' emotional state and being sympathetic and aligned to how they're feeling will allow you to improve the service for them.

VALUE

When it comes to service, it's not about price. What's important is that the service you deliver matches the value of whatever the customer hands over, however large or small of an amount that is. You can raise the value that you offer in your service by going above and beyond, by delighting and surprising your clients. When you do that, that's when your customer feels like they've had an amazing, valuable service and they feel that, whatever they're spending, they have got value for money.

This isn't about whether your prices are cheaper or more expensive than somewhere else, this is about whether your customers feel that they get value for money from your service. You want customers to be shopping based on the value rather than the price of your services. Then it doesn't really matter how much you charge, as long as every customer feels that they are getting value for money.

Many salon owners make the mistake of believing that people shop on price alone, but that's not true. Let's say that there's one salon offering a cut and blow dry to new customers for £35, which is a traditional cut, design, shampoo and blow dry, and then you leave the salon and you're done. Just down the road is another salon that's offering a cut and blow dry for £50. Many salon owners will think that the customer will automatically go for the cheaper option.

But what if when that customer enquires about the £50 cut and blow dry they're told that, as a new customer, they'll get a full consultation with a stylist, that the salon only uses premium products and will advise you on the best products for your hair? They're also told that they'll get a complimentary conditioning treatment worth £10 and, when they leave, they get to take home a goody bag containing vouchers and a free shampoo worth £10. All of a sudden, that extra £15 feels like excellent value for money. That's not to say that the other salon, where a cut is £35, wouldn't have done some or even all of those things, but the point is that they haven't told the customer that. Also the cost of the free shampoo can be minimal if you make a deal with your supplier, and the vouchers in the goody bag encourage the returns we want.

There are plenty of other ways that you can add value to someone's experience, such as offering a complimentary head or hand massage and making sure the complimentary refreshments you serve are of a really high standard.

At my salon we send out birthday cards to all of our clients. At Easter we give customers a little Easter egg to take home with them, as well as many other changing treats. It's those small surprises that just delight people and it's those small touches that people remember. That's what adding value to service is all about.

INFORM

This also ties in with what I talked about under educate, where you're managing client expectations. Inform is all about making sure your clients know what all of your policies are, especially cancellation policies, and being clear about your terms and conditions. This is a really important part of the service because if you haven't fully informed people about terms and conditions and those little details, it's very easy to disappoint them. Then it won't matter if you've given them great service, because what they'll remember is that feeling of disappointment.

You should also make sure you inform your clients about any deals or offers that you've got in your salon. This is about allowing every one of your customers to make an informed choice about what products, packages or services they buy from you. It's really important that all of your stylists and therapists do this too, otherwise one person might overhear another client being given all this information and wonder why it's not being shared with them too, which will have a negative impact on their experience.

CARE

Care is just everything bundled up. Customer care is exactly what it says: it's not about the initial transaction and money coming in, it's about truly caring about your customers and whether they can look after their hair at home. I talked about informing people about how to look after their hair, such as how to take care of their colour, but this is about caring that if you don't do that part of your job, if you don't inform them, then they could wash £100–£200 worth of colour down the drain.

It's also caring about your team and the environment you create at your salon. That's all part of the service you provide and really this step is just thinking about a customer's journey, and taking care at every step, to make sure they're getting what they want.

It's important to recognise that all of the elements – your customers, your team and your business – are interlinked. Without customers, you won't have a business and you won't need a team. Without your team, you can't serve your customers. If your business isn't doing well, you won't have a team or customers. They are all equally important because none would exist without the other.

At my salon, we very much have a partnership mentality, in that we really care about our customers and we never look down on anyone because they don't understand the technicalities of what we can and can't do with their hair. This ties back in with education and making sure that, as the professionals, you're explaining what is and isn't possible to your customers.

Your business has to have a heart and customer care needs to be right at the centre of that. The people in your team need to align with that too, otherwise your customers will feel it.

Care is also about putting the customer first. If you're serving them and you're not telling them about the offers you have available or the retail products they should be taking home to look after their hair or skin etc., then you're putting yourself and often your own fears first. You're not putting the customer first.

Truly caring about the customer can often help members of the team to get over the fear they have around sharing offers or talking about retail products because they know that if they really care about their customer, they will educate and inform them. You have to remind them that it's not about them, their fears or whatever is going on in their heads, it's about the customer and giving them what they want and need. That's what's at the heart of caring.

ELEVATE

This is about knowing that you've elevated your customers in some way after each and every interaction they have with you. What you want is that, regardless of the stage in their journey, your customers feel elevated. It doesn't matter whether they've seen your website for the first time, made an enquiry, booked an appointment, come in for their first visit or had their 1,000th appointment, you want them to leave your salon feeling good about themselves.

You might achieve that through conversation, the value you provide, your immaculate service or the feeling in the salon. One thing that's very important is that you always highlight what's good about your client. Too many professionals will focus on the negative and say things like, 'Your hair's really dry.' Of course there are things that need to be fixed, that's why the customer is there, but you should be mindful of what's good about them and draw their attention to that.

Your customer will probably tell you about the areas that need work during the consultation, so make sure you find things that are good and mention those. Their hair might be dry, but you could make a comment like, 'Your hair's really thick and strong.' If all you do is focus on the areas that need to be fixed, you'll knock their confidence and they won't leave the salon feeling elevated.

I think sometimes professionals can forget how that can make people feel and focus too much on the problems.

My advice is to encourage the customer to lead the consultation and really listen to them. They will know the problems they have with their hair and they'll tell you. A great question to ask is, 'How do you feel about your hair at the moment?' Their answer to that question will show you where they are and your job is to elevate them from that level. You want them to leave feeling better not worse.

My favourite sales question is, 'What is important to you about X?' Just fill in the X with whatever service you offer, for example hair, skin or nails. Then the client will start to tell you what they value the most, which helps you offer aftercare as the solution to their issues. This is called consultative sales.

Give your customers compliments. You can always find something good about someone. It might be that they have beautiful shoes on or a lovely coat. If you think that when they walk in, don't keep it to yourself, tell them. Also don't underestimate the importance of calling your customers by their name and the effect that can have.

For me, listening is the thread that runs through the whole customer journey and ends with elevating each customer. People want to feel heard and seen, so make sure you really listen to what they're saying. Listening is a vital part of your communication. Focus on your customer and do everything you can to make sure they leave you feeling better than when they walked into your salon.

'Good Salon Guide was proud to award Salon Jedi Academy with a 5 Star Good Training Guide, the first ever for a digital training platform and it's a fantastic platform for business owners to take advantage of Caroline's hard-won, and proven, business and marketing advice.'

- ***Gareth Penn, Director, GSG***

CASE STUDY
LISA PHILLIPS

My name is Lisa Phillips and I run Ora Hair in Banstead. Before I started training with Caroline at Salon Jedi, I'd grown my business a little, but I felt it had plateaued. I was struggling to get to the next level and I knew I needed help.

At this stage my salon was making a small profit, but we definitely weren't maximising the business at all. My biggest problem was that I was still working in the business rather than on the business. I was having fear issues about taking myself off the shop floor, which meant I was juggling my time between running a column, doing the training, managing and motivating my team, and generally running the business. I've always done mindset coaching with my team, but at this point I didn't have the time to keep on top of it and we got stuck.

I needed to have more confidence in myself that I was doing the right thing in coming off the floor and focusing more on marketing the business and supporting my team. However, I felt guilty about coming off the floor. I thought that by running my column, I was being a good influence and I worried that if I left that behind, I wouldn't be such a good influence on my team. As well as being a hairdresser, I've also trained as a yoga teacher and I felt like I was struggling to bring that calming influence into my business.

Looking for help

At the end of the summer of 2019, I realised I needed help. I was firefighting all the time. I felt like I had a great team, but I also felt like I was letting them down because I wasn't able to support them as much as they needed.

It was at this point that a post about an event Caroline was running popped up in my newsfeed on Facebook. I decided to go along to her summit and her story really resonated with me. Everything she'd done and implemented was what I was trying to do. She'd been where I was and I could see that everything she'd talked about, she'd implemented, which was different to some of the other business trainers I'd worked with or listened to before.

Following the right path

The first thing I had to do when I started working with Caroline was get over that guilt and realise how much I was getting in my own way. As I was going through her online training, it was ticking boxes in my own head. I found myself thinking, 'Yes, you are on the right path. What you're trying to implement is working for someone else.'

As I've gone through the course, it's just clarified for me that I am on the right path. I've also found the support of the rest of the group incredibly valuable. It gives you accountability and it really helps to feel like you're part of a network of people who understand. Every time you make changes and you see positive results, it just confirms that you're on the right path.

Changes that lead to results

When I started training with Caroline, I had put systems in place at my salon and I thought I'd broken them down into smaller parts and smaller parts, but I hadn't. This made me strip back everything I had in my systems and really get down to the nitty gritty of it all. I went into much smaller details – now I've got systems for systems!

This has been a really good exercise because it's helped me go into the much smaller details, but it's also helped me see how everything works together as part of the big picture.

Quieting my doubts

When I was running my business before I joined Caroline's course, I would often wonder whether I was expecting too much of my team, or too much of my manager or my receptionist. The great thing with Caroline's training is that you can see that everything she's telling you to do – or not do – is working for them. When you can see that Caroline and Carla are doing everything they're telling you to do, and that it's working, it gives you the confidence to implement it yourself. I've certainly taken this on board and implemented their training in my salon and it's working for me too.

The biggest change I've made is taking myself off the shop floor. The lockdown in the UK that came about because of the Covid-19 pandemic came at a really good time for me, shortly after I'd started my training. Just like every other salon, we had to close for three months and since we opened back up in July 2020, I haven't seen any clients at all. I've been managing my business from my home. This period has really made me delegate all my jobs to other members of my team in my salon and now I'm really utilising every one of my team members.

By giving them jobs and accountability, it's allowed me to have time to really market my business. Before, I didn't have time to focus on marketing my business, or to analyse the marketing we were doing. Stepping out of the salon has also given me time to work on myself and do my own training, whereas before I didn't have the time or energy to do that.

Now I know that I'm not asking too much of my team, and I think they feel more empowered and happier because not only do they have more jobs to do, but they're clear about what their jobs are and they know that I trust them. I'll freely admit that before I was a bit of a control freak, but having that guidance from Caroline has helped me to get off the shop floor and work from behind the scenes.

Focusing on staff training

During lockdown I made sure all the members of my team did Caroline's mindful training course called the Mindful Salon Source Code. I felt that I'd already managed to employ the right team, so this period just gave me a chance to implement the training I wanted to do with them but that I'd previously struggled to make time for. Now they know where I'm coming from, which means I can give them a task and I know they're doing it with my values in place, which means they're making the right choices. That makes them happier because they feel like I trust them because I'm not being so controlling, and I'm happier because I know I can trust my team.

Seeing the results

At the time of writing in 2020, we've only been able to open and serve customers properly in January, February and July. In those three months, we've made just over £9,000 more than what we need to make, just by implementing some of the things that Caroline has taught me. Those extra sales are just from up-serves as a result of the changes we've made. In just three months of work, two of which being typically quieter (January and February), I've already made a return on the course investment with upgrades alone. Caroline and the Salon Jedi team also created a beautiful new website for me during lockdown, which is already number one on Google and sending me new clients.

I would tell anyone who's in the position I was in a year ago, where you're struggling to get off the shop floor and run your business rather than being in your business, to do the course. You will make your money back and even if you only make your money back and nothing more, you haven't lost anything.

For me, improving my management has been about a lot more than money. It's given me a better lifestyle, made me less stressed and given me more time. I've gained all of this, and lots more, just by listening to somebody who's already implemented what I wanted to do. Six months after joining the Salon Jedi Academy, I am now off the tools – I'm the owner working ON the business, not IN it.

ARE YOU STRUGGLING TO MANAGE YOUR TEAM? IF YOU WOULD LIKE TO BOOK A FREE BREAKTHROUGH DISCOVERY CALL, SCAN THE QR CODE BELOW USING YOUR MOBILE PHONE'S CAMERA AND SELECT THE TIME THAT WORKS FOR YOU.

This breakthrough call is to look inside your business to see how to improve profits, scalability and leverage, and to identify any limiting beliefs holding you back.

We will help you discover what is not working in your salon business and plan how to scale up and reach your dream profits, even while getting off the tools if you wish.

PART 4

MAINTENANCE

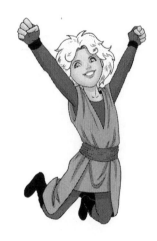

Do you remember our salon owners from Part 1 of the book? We had Sandra who was stuck in a fixed mindset and Jenny who had a growth mindset. We're going to take a look at how Jenny is getting on three years later.

REVISITING JENNY...

Jenny feels frazzled. The salon has been busy all day and she feels like she's barely stopped. She walks into the back office and flops into the chair at her desk, sighing as she sits. Even though she has a bigger salon and more stylists, she doesn't feel like she's making headway.

She leans forward and puts her head in her hands, *What a day!* There were two customer complaints today. They're the fifth and sixth this week. One wasn't happy with the cut they received from the new stylist and the other was upset she couldn't use her free blow dry voucher on a Saturday. *I know our standards are slipping but I don't know what to do! We're just too busy to cope with all these customers.* Jenny lifts her head out of her hands, takes a deep breath and composes herself. *Where did I go wrong? I thought I was doing everything right to grow my business.*

Just then there's a knock at the door and her manager's head appears. 'Just bringing you the figures and takings for today,' she says. 'Thank you,' Jenny says with a wan smile. She doesn't stay for a chat. Jenny feels bad that she didn't make more of an effort but she just doesn't have the energy. As she inputs the figures into her spreadsheet, she can see that although they've been busy, they're not making much more than their expenses. *I can't put my prices up, can I? Surely I'll lose all my customers! But I'm already losing customers.*

The thought lingers, niggling in the corner of her brain. She knows that it's true. There have been several regulars who haven't been back for months, but she can't quite put her finger on what it is that's turning them away. She decides to call it a day, she has a meeting with her accountant on Monday and she needs to prepare. *There goes Sunday afternoon!* she thinks as she turns off her computer and gets ready to leave.

When Jenny arrives at her accountant's office on Monday morning, she's offered a cup of tea. It's too hot to drink, so she holds it, warming up her hands after being out in the cold. She has her latest figures in her bag, even though she probably won't need them for this meeting. She has a knot in her stomach and it's refusing to shift. She takes a sip of her tea, almost burning her tongue.

Sitting in her accountant's office, facing him across the desk, she tries her best to smile. 'Do you want the good news or the bad news first?' he says. *Oh god.* 'The good news?' Jenny says hesitantly. He smiles. 'Well, this tax year you've turned over more than ever before...' Jenny feels the knot easing, she breaks into a smile. 'Really?' *It's felt like such hard work though.* 'Yes, your turnover is up £35,000. However...' *Here it comes.* The knot is back and this time it definitely feels bigger than before. 'Your costs have increased significantly by over £50,000 so your net profits are down again.' Jenny feels like her stomach has fallen through the floor. She stares intently at her tea, watching the steam rise out of the cup. She wants to scream, 'But why am I not making any money when I work so hard?'

As she leaves her accountant, she wants to cry. She barely held it together in the meeting. *How did this happen? How did I not realise we were spending this much?* Jenny feels out of her depth. It's not just that the world of hairdressing seems to be changing around her, but that she's losing her grasp on her salon. She doesn't feel excited to go into work every day any more and she doesn't remember when that changed. With a heavy heart and a sick feeling in her stomach, she walks down the cold street towards her salon. The wind whips around the corner and looking up she can see grey clouds gathering thick and fast. *How am I going to turn this around?'*

When we first met Jenny she was doing well with her growth mindset and had a clear vision for her salon and where she wanted to take the business. She was passionate about hairdressing and that helped her grow and helped her attract the right people to her small team.

However, in subsequent years she's become a victim of her own success, and her mindset work went by the wayside as she got busier and busier. I often encounter salon owners who have started well but who haven't had the systems in place to maintain their standards and their early success. Failing to have a solid foundation in place is what's resulted in Jenny taking home less and less money each year for herself. She's started running her business from a place of fear, where she's scared to charge more. She's taken her eye off the ball, which is how she's gone over her expenses without realising. She's not investing in training herself or her staff, which is why the standards at her salon are slipping. She doesn't have the time to work on marketing, which is why she's struggling to attract new customers.

This final part of the book explores the maintenance side of your business. I'm going to explain systems and why having these in place is so important as you get busier. Things will start to implode if you don't have a solid foundation. This comes back to knowing your core values and focusing on those. The trouble is, when things start to go wrong, it becomes very easy to slip back into a fixed mindset where all you see is problems. That pushes you into a downward spiral and if you lose sight of your mission and your purpose it will drag you down.

In this part of the book, I'm going to talk to you about creating a culture within your business that focuses on your core values. Having this culture and being very clear about your mission and your vision is revolutionary – it certainly was for me. This is what defines the most successful businesses in any industry. They're the ones that stand out and they're the ones that get things done, even when it looks like it might be crumbling. That's because they have such a strong foundation to lean back on.

I'll also explain systems and automation, which is essential for time management and helping you to spend more time off the floor managing the business. It's the systems that you put in place that provide that strong core. Measuring and tracking your numbers is another essential element to get right when it comes to maintenance, because it's this that will prevent you from having any nasty surprises like an unexpected VAT bill, which happened to me back in my dark days. I had gone over the VAT threshold without knowing and found out I owed £11,000... ouch!

Finally, I'm going to talk briefly about scaling to exit your business. There's a clear distinction to make between being a business operator and being a business owner. If you want to exit your business, or have the option of exiting your business, you need to show prospective buyers that it isn't reliant on you in order to make it more attractive and get the best possible price for it. Operator-run businesses will get less as YOU are the business and when you sell you leave with the sale. This is why managed businesses that don't rely on the owner as the operator, and that have systems in place, are worth way more at sale. All of the other elements of maintenance feed into this, but the systems and automation are particularly useful when it comes to scaling. If you get all of this in place then if you want to scale you can scale, and if you want to exit you can exit.

If you implement everything I'm going to talk about in the coming chapters, as well as what I've already spoken about, this will not only make your business more efficient, create leverage and give you more time, it will also make your business more valuable.

CHAPTER 12

CREATING A CULTURE

Nowadays people like to buy from companies or people that have a mission, are authentic and that are driven by a bigger purpose and have values. That's why people predominantly buy from people that they like and trust. When you have a mission statement that's clear about your core values and purpose, it attracts your tribe.

Creating a culture with these core values at its heart has a number of benefits beyond this, and that's why identifying your core values and your purpose is one of the first things we train our Salon Jedi students in. When you have these core values, it makes it easier to run your salon. Your decisions are based around them, your staff will follow them and you'll recruit people who are aligned with those values.

'I have always dreamed of a salon that had five star customer service, a team that worked together and towards becoming better and better in hairdressing skills and personal development, and a business that ran with systems and procedures.

We have found all this in the education that comes from Caroline and the Salon Jedi team. They have helped us discover who we are, what we are about, where we are going and helped us to dream again in our business.'

- **Darren Mitzi, Darren Michael Hairdressing**

MAKE DECISIONS THAT SUPPORT YOUR CULTURE

Your core values are especially important when it comes to decision making. I often see salon owners getting a little bit lost because they're making emotional decisions in the moment, rather than making a decision that's supported by their core values and that therefore supports the culture they've created. As I said in an earlier chapter, your core values are what gives you the inner strength to step in and correct behaviour that doesn't align with your culture, or to make decisions on pricing regardless of what your competitors are doing.

I'm always happy to listen to my team if they have any suggestions or if they want to ask me for anything, but my decision will always be based on our culture. The core values are the first things I think of. My salon is a partnership that's centred around the business, the team and the clients. Before I make any decision, I have to ask myself what is in the best interests of the company, the team and the clients.

For example, let's say a stylist asks me if they can take a holiday in December. I'll ask myself if this is the best decision for everybody and the answer will be 'No'. It's not in the best interests of the clients, because December is a really busy month so if one stylist takes a week off we'll be able to serve fewer clients. It's not in the best interests of the team, because they'll be under more pressure because there will be fewer staff members in. And as a result of both of those, it's not in the best interests of the business. It's not an emotional decision and it's not based on favouritism, it's one that is based purely on our culture. It has to be, because if you're prepared to say yes to a request like that for one person, then you have to be prepared to say yes to everybody.

LIVE BY YOUR CORE VALUES

You have to make sure that not only your team but also your clients see that you're living up to your core values and your culture. If you're saying that something is a core value, but then your actions go against that, your team and your clients will see that and it breaks their trust in you and it lowers your integrity.

It's also important to consider your culture when you're setting goals and when you're making decisions that lead towards one of your goals. For example, you might have a goal of owning a chain of five salons, but you have to make sure that you're in a strong enough position with a strong enough culture that this can be replicated in your next salon. Otherwise you could lose some of your core values, and therefore your integrity, along the way.

This is particularly important if you're opening a new salon, because you can't be everywhere. You have to think very carefully about who's going to manage the culture in your new salon and who is going to make sure that everyone at your new location is, and stays, aligned to your core values. It's all well and good to train any new staff members when they first come in, but you also need to have someone there to maintain the values and make sure that your culture runs across your salons. That's true whether you're going to the new salon to get it up and running, in which case you need to have someone to maintain the culture in your existing salon, or whether you're bringing someone in to run your new salon for you.

Maintenance of the culture is so important to ensure that it doesn't get diluted as you multiply and to make sure that you keep that culture alive across the whole business.

UNDERSTAND WHAT YOU HAVE TO DO TO MAINTAIN YOUR CORE VALUES

You need to know what's required to maintain your core values. For example, at my salon one of our core values is to be in the top 10% of salons in the UK. If we want to maintain that as part of our culture, we have to keep training the team, we have to stay on the pulse of what's new in the industry, we need to keep entering awards and we need to keep being seen.

That's an example of how our core values and our culture filter through into our decision making and behaviour at the business.

MAKE SURE YOU MAINTAIN NEW IDEAS LONG ENOUGH TO BECOME PART OF THE CULTURE

One issue I often see in salons is that the salon owner has a great idea about how to do something differently. Let's use retail as an example. A salon owner creates a wonderful new system for their retail, where their team consult their customers and then offer them three retail products and really focus on advising the customers on what's best for them.

The salon owner holds a team meeting to explain the new system and new approach to retail. She might even bring in an educator to help explain the concept that we talked about in the sales chapter, about how retail is advising, not selling. Everyone is buzzing and for the first couple of weeks the new system is working really well, but then it starts to drop off, and it's not only the sales that start to drop but the targets too. Staff members are reluctant to do it because they see that other people on the team aren't following the system. What has happened is that this new system wasn't maintained for long enough for it to become embedded in the culture of the salon.

This maintenance is key and it's why this part of the book is so important. It's about more than running one training session and feeling as though you've ticked that box. It's about continually training staff and correcting them when they don't follow the new system so that this culture, this way of doing things, gets programmed into their minds. Once you install this culture at an individual level, it naturally becomes part of daily life in the salon.

YOU HAVE TO MAINTAIN YOUR CULTURE

There's a very strong culture at my salon, but the reason it is strong and has stayed strong for so many years is that we maintain it. We constantly remind everyone of how important our culture is. We make sure that we keep training around our culture and supporting the team. We make sure that we're updating our culture. And we make sure that we're putting it all into practice. If we didn't do all of those things, our culture would soon morph into something new with diluted standards.

If you neglect your culture, then no matter how strong it is, it will start to slide, much like standards do. What you have to remember is that it's much easier to maintain a culture and keep it going than it is to build a new one from scratch. It's like spinning plates, they just need a little spin to keep them going.

YOU HAVE A CULTURE, WHETHER YOU KNOW IT OR NOT

Even if you've never consciously thought about the culture in your salon, you have one. That culture might be that the staff can do what they want, or that your staff make up the rules and as the owner you're too scared to challenge them. Whatever you're doing, both with your team and your service, that's your culture.

If you're realising that you have a culture like this, don't panic. You can change it, but you have to change it to a culture that you want and make it one where people can thrive. When you do this, you'll find that you start to attract more of what you want and you'll have the awareness and strength to say no to what you don't want.

YOUR CULTURE IS YOUR CORE

This is a very simple concept, but it's really important that you get the right culture embedded in your salon if you want to grow your business. This culture is the core that you can build upon. If you don't have a strong culture at the core of your salon, you'll start to see problems as you expand.

If you're busy and you're growing so you decide to open a second salon, and then maybe a third, you'll start to see the weakness in your foundations if you haven't created this strong core culture to support you and your business as you expand. If your culture isn't strong enough, or maybe you aren't as consciously aware of your culture as you need to be, you can start to hire the wrong people into the business and, as it grows, it becomes more challenging to manage and maintain your business.

OUR HAPPINESS CULTURE

At my salon, part of our culture is a happiness culture. It's positivity. To align with that, when you walk into the salon you'll see positive messages around. When our clients leave, we'll give them a little scroll with a positive message on it. We might even send them a text containing a positive message. It's very much about lifting people's vibrations and elevating them.

For example, during the Covid-19 lockdown we sent a text message telling our clients how valued they are and missed. We created a 'we miss you' video, and our NHS clap video was automatically posted on our Facebook wall at 8pm every Thursday. We also held an Easter egg competition and ran quizzes. We also offered free chats with our team for anyone feeling down or lonely.

Being positive is very important to us and it's why we're so careful about who we hire into our team. We're happy for someone to come in who maybe isn't that positive, but who wants to become more positive. However, we aren't going to hire somebody who isn't aligned with the positivity in our culture and who has no interest in changing, because when you bring in someone like that, their energy can start to infect others and, before you know it, your team start to get more and more negative and unhappy. We have built our happiness culture and we all work together to maintain and protect it.

CHAPTER 13

SYSTEMS AND AUTOMATION

As a salon owner myself, I can admit that the idea of systems and automation doesn't excite me. I'm a creative person, as are you I imagine, which is why we went into this field. However, one thing that does excite me, and that I'm sure excites you, is having more freedom; and like me you may want to reduce or remove your time from the tools. Systems and automation are essential for giving you that freedom and time, but you can't have one without the other.

Of course there will be some of you who love structure and who are excited about this chapter, which is great. However you feel about the idea of systems and automation, it's important to understand that you need to put systems in place to make your salon run more smoothly and to automate more tasks, which in turn will free up your time. Systemisation and automation also helps to add value to your business, as I mentioned earlier, which is essential if you want to have the option of exiting, which I'll talk more about in the final chapter.

EXERCISE

WHAT DO SYSTEMS GIVE YOU MORE AND LESS OF?

I'm going to give you some examples of what systems can give you more of, and I'll also give you some examples of what systems can give you less of. Underneath each of these sections is a space where you can write down any other things that you think systems will give you more or less of.

Systems give you more...

- Freedom – you can get off the tools.
- Clarity – everyone knows where they stand.
- Time – when you start automating you get time to spend on other tasks.
- Direction.
- Security – if you go through systems as part of your induction process, you'll know that new starts have covered everything they need to know.

Systems give you less...

- Stress.
- Grey areas – staff all know what the procedures and policies are.
- Chaos.
- Customer complaints.

YOU CAN DUPLICATE SYSTEMS

Once you have a system that works, you can duplicate that for other areas of your business. Duplication also applies to training. When you have systems in place, it makes your induction process really easy. You can see exactly what's been done because you have everything on a checklist and you tick those off and get your new team member to sign it to say they've covered it.

WHAT SHOULD BE SYSTEMISED?

The short answer to that is absolutely everything! What you're doing with your systems is documenting how you like things to be done in your salon. These documents don't have to be long and complicated, they can be as simple as a photo or a video, as long as it is documented and easily consumable to the team.

If you've got a new Saturday assistant starting, you can say, 'This is how we serve our teas and coffees' and show them a photo of how you like them to be presented; or, 'This is how we fold our towels' and again, show them a photo of how they should be folded. You don't have to spend time actually doing those things with them, because you've got a really simple visual reference that they can look at and copy. All you have to do is put those photos together in a folder in the salon. It's that simple. Systems don't have to be rocket science.

Your systems should document how you do everything, from how you answer the phone to how you greet clients when they come into the salon. Include a copy of your client journey. You can make specific system manuals for different parts of your salon too, such as having a reception manual for your front of house team to refer to.

You can also make your systems documents as long or short as you want and you can call them whatever you want. We call ours the Ego Operating System. Our operations manual has been adapted for availability to our Salon Jedi Academy students. Just contact us if you need any help with this (you'll find our contact details at the end of the book).

WHY ARE SYSTEMS SO IMPORTANT?

Systems ensure that every member of your team knows how things should be done and that everyone does things in the same way. If everyone on your team isn't doing everything in the same way, the customer experience becomes diluted.

One of the biggest mistakes salons make is not teaching new members of staff how you do things at your salon. What happens then is that this new person does things differently, and if no one does anything about it then, all of a sudden, your culture, and the way you want things to be done, changes. This might just start with one person, but it will filter through to other members of the team until suddenly you find yourself saying, 'We used to do that.'

It's especially important to put systems in place and make sure that they're followed if one of your aims is to get off the salon floor. Otherwise what can happen is that you walk into your salon after two or maybe three months of not being there so much and you find that things have moved or processes have changed and it's not the way you want it to be any more.

> '[Caroline] is a visionary with some of the most incredible ideas, she is driven and has enjoyed well-deserved success as a result. Straight talking and results motivated – every salon needs Caroline in their life to help them take control and propel their own business forward.'
>
> -   **Sally Learmouth, Director, Gloss Communications**

INDUCTIONS ARE REALLY IMPORTANT

This is why inductions for new staff are so important, because you need to make sure that they know what your systems are and that they follow them. We always have a full induction day with any new member of staff. They watch training videos, they read whatever documents they need to read, and you tick off and document everything you've taught them and shown them on a checklist.

AUTOMATE AS MUCH AS YOU CAN

I always say that everything should be systemised, but if you can automate it then that's even better. I love automation because it gives me time back.

At my salon we have automated text reminders for appointments, we run automated text marketing (as I mentioned in the marketing part of the book) and everything on our website is automated using an auto responder. That means if someone signs up for their welcome voucher, the auto responder will send out continued communication, which helps me build that relationship with a new client. Automated messenger bots are another tool that you should invest in. I've met a lot of salon owners who have clients sending them messages through their Messenger page at 11 or 12 at night, enquiring about appointments. Even though they complain about it, they'll feel obliged to reply. Whereas if they use a messenger bot, that can direct clients to online bookings, packages, marketing or even answer frequently asked questions, depending on what the client says. This frees up their time.

We also have an automated call manager service, which means that whenever someone calls the salon they'll never hear an engaged tone. They'll get an automated message telling them they'll be put on hold until we can answer their call, and while they're waiting they'll hear our marketing messages. With this system, if we do miss a call for any reason, that person receives an automated text message saying, 'Sorry we missed your call, we're going to call you straight back.' This reduces the chances of them trying somewhere else.

Automation doesn't just have to mean using technology. You can also automate things like marketing through your team by way of automatic responses and systems. This comes back to systemising activity and having processes in place, like I talked about in the marketing part of the book, where sending out the letters to the new clients from the week before happens every Monday morning at my salon, for example.

AUTOMATION FOR YOUR MANAGEMENT

Automation isn't just for dealing with customers and making sure that you provide the best service possible. It's also useful for me to keep on top of how the salon is running. For example, I get a text message each night telling me how many calls the salon received during the day and how many of those were missed. Having everything in the salon computerised is also really useful because that allows me to log in and check everything, from how much we've spent on stock to how much we've taken and how the marketing is performing.

Because I'm working from home and I'm not in the salon all the time, this is incredibly valuable for me. It means I'm always aware of what's going on in the salon, even if I'm not physically there. When you're smart with your systems and automation, you can have eyes on, and get feedback from, not just one, but potentially multiple salons.

SYSTEMS DON'T HAVE TO BE OVERWHELMING

When you start looking at systems and how you can introduce them, I know that it might seem overwhelming, but instead of worrying about all the parts that need to be systemised and monitored, think of it as one big folder that is your operating system, with lots of subfolders within it that are for each of the areas of your business, such as stock, recruitment, inductions, staff, reception and so on. Within those subfolders there are 'how to' files for each of the systems. This helps you chunk it down and deal with one thing at a time. It's also a really good way of organising your operating system and making it logical, as this is how the brain works and will help you find what you need.

It's also important to make the distinction between processes and procedures. Processes are the 'why' and the procedure is the 'how'. Each of your systems should include both of these elements.

CHAPTER 14

MEASURING AND TRACKING YOUR NUMBERS

Knowing your numbers and maintaining your figures is an essential part of maintenance. Business is all about numbers. Everything in your business has a number and every member of your team should have a number.

You should start by working out your big numbers. Those are your breakeven and your target. From there, you work out what each team member's targets are. When you look at the most successful businesses and companies in the world, they all have clear goals and everyone has a number that they're working towards. This is how it should be in your salon.

For example, if you've got a stylist or therapist who's working towards being promoted to senior level, there will be a number that they've got to hit to reach that level if you're working on a tier-level system, for instance. These are what are called your KPIs (key performance indicators) for things such as percentage of rebooking and retail.

CHUNK DOWN YOUR NUMBERS

Remember in Chapters 2 and 6 when I talked about setting your big goals and how you have to chunk them down to the ridiculous? It's no different with numbers. Come back to this idea of having one big folder, which represents your big number, and within that are subfolders, which are all of the steps along the way to hitting that big number.

For example, if you have a three-year target, break it down so that you know what that looks like per year, per quarter, per month, per week, per day, per morning, per afternoon, per hour, per stylist or therapist. This is an exercise in understanding: you need to break your numbers down to the extent that you know what each team member needs to take extra in a day for you to hit that big figure.

HOW DO YOU SERVE UP YOUR PIE?

This also allows you to work out the optimum percentage that you should spend on marketing, stock and your expenses like rent and bills. Think back to Chapter 6, where I talked about revenue and how you only have one pie. You need to divide that pie up and know exactly what portion of it is for stock, what portion is for wages, rent, sundries and of course net profits. You cut the profits portion of your pie first, and only then can you budget all your other expenses.

What happens all too often is that salon owners don't keep track of how they're carving up their pie. They give it out to all their expenses first and then realise there is nothing left for themselves. How can you thrive when you're starving yourself?

In the early days of running a business, you might have fewer people to feed from your pie, but you'll also have a smaller pie from which to feed them. Often what happens in the early days of a business is that you start borrowing pieces from other people's pies.

As I mentioned in Chapter 6, it's crucial that you understand that if you give a bigger slice of pie to one area, you have to take it from another. For example, if the percentage of your pie that you spend on wages goes over by 10%, you have to take that from another area. If you can't find that money from another area of your budget, it's going to come from your net profit. If you take too much from your net profit then your business fails to be profitable.

You can see an example of our numbers and how we serve up our pie by following the QR code below.

MY STORY

YOUR BUSINESS PLAN ISN'T JUST FOR YOUR BANK

When I started my business, I worked with someone who really knew business to create my business plan. He helped me create my business plan and I took this to the bank. Now, this business plan was so tight with the figures and expenses and I thought I'd covered everything, but the fact was there wasn't much left after all these things. The mistake I made, and I imagine I'm not the only person who has done this, was that I created my business plan to take to the bank to get the funds I needed to start my business; I didn't create my business plan to understand my numbers.

Once I'd got my funds from the bank, I didn't really look at that business plan again and I didn' t even try to follow it. I don't remember a lot of what was in that business plan, but what I do remember is that I received a £10,000 loan to start my business and in the business plan I predicted that I'd make £52,000 in profit by year five. The reality was by year five I made £52,000 in turnover and almost went bankrupt. That just goes to show why it's so important to know your figures.

When I opened my business I knew nothing about the figures. I just opened my salon with a couple of chair renters and thought that their rent would cover the expenses and then I'd be able to take whatever came in over that, but all these random expenses that I hadn't factored in kept popping up. That was especially true when I started employing people and I realised I had to pay employer contributions. I really did learn on the job and that's very similar for a lot of salon owners.

I hadn't set aside a budget for marketing; in fact I didn't even know what marketing really meant and I didn't understand it. I didn't know anything about KPIs, I didn't have a computer system and I didn't track anything except my takings. I'd get my year-end figures but I wouldn't have a clue what they meant. I just winged it at the beginning, but it was when I started to employ people that things began to unravel and I ended up on the verge of bankruptcy. This was the point at which I realised I needed to look more closely at my figures, because I needed to work out how much I could afford to pay people and what every aspect of my business was costing me.

WHY UNDERSTANDING YOUR NUMBERS IS SO IMPORTANT

Understanding your numbers isn't just about knowing your breakeven, your staffing costs and your expenses, although these are all important. It's also about understanding how much you need to grow, how much you need to budget for marketing and what targets you're trying to hit.

When you don't have a clear view of all of these elements, your business isn't built on a strong foundation. It's weak and it's vulnerable. That means as soon as there's any kind of downturn, all your blind spots will be exposed and you'll start to struggle.

NUMBERS AREN'T JUST FINANCES

There are many figures within your business that you should be tracking (KPIs) and be aware of if you want to be successful. They include, but are not limited to:

- The number of clients you have coming through your doors.
- What percentage are rebooking.
- The percentages of customers booking for the various services you offer.
- The percentage you're making on retail compared to services.
- Average bill size.

LOOKING BEYOND THE NUMBERS

Some salon owners might already be tracking these numbers, setting targets and KPIs for their staff and chunking down their figures to an extent, but they might not know how to move the business forward.

For instance, they could be setting targets for their staff but if they're not bringing enough customers through the doors of the salon, their team won't be able to hit those targets. Or it might be that two of their top-earning members of staff leave or take maternity leave within a short period of each other and all of a sudden they have a gaping hole in their income that they hadn't allowed for. It could also be that the salon owner is focused on their goal of opening four or five salons and they scale too quickly, without the systems and figures in place to support it.

The problem with that is that, if there's any weakness in your business, as you grow the weakness grows with it. What might have been manageable in one salon suddenly becomes unmanageable in two or three. It's not sustainable and it's not secure.

'Two days after [Caroline and Carla] left the salon, we saw a 261% increase in sales because we implemented the changes they had put in place. Then sales increased the next month by £1,000, then £2,000 the month after that and kept growing.'

- ***Amanda Allan, Heavenly Sensations***

IT'S ALL ABOUT BALANCE

There is no one-size-fits-all when it comes to the percentage that you should be spending on wages, stock, marketing and so on. I can't give you that because every salon is different. What I can tell you is that everything needs to be balanced. What you have coming in needs to be more than what you have going out. It's no good growing the size of your pie if the size of the slices you're giving away grows more than the pie does.

It's also important not to get too hung up on the percentage of the pie that you're taking. If you've got a small pie and are taking 40% of it, that might mean you're not earning as much money as if you've got a much bigger pie and are taking 25% of it. There are so many variables you have to consider and these will be unique to your business.

EXAMPLE: SMALLER PERCENTAGES DON'T NECESSARILY MEAN LESS MONEY

To explain this, imagine that you have a stylist who's bringing in £1,000 a week and they're being paid 30% of whatever they bring in. That means they're earning £300 a week.

At another salon, you might have a stylist who's only getting paid 25% of whatever they bring in, but in a week they're bringing in £2,000, which means they get paid £500.

This is why it's so important to look at the figures based on your salon and nowhere else. A salon that spends a lot of money and time on marketing, awards and training might only offer their stylists 30% of their takings, but if that marketing spend means they're bringing in higher figures, financially the stylists will be better off than those who are working at a salon where they get 40% of their weekly takings, but they have fewer appointments so they're only getting 40% of £800, for example.

It's important that you, as the salon owner, can communicate the value you add for your stylists and explain these figures to them.

HOW TO START MEASURING AND TRACKING YOUR NUMBERS

You have to start by simplifying everything. Begin by calculating the breakeven costs you have to spend in order to function before you employ anyone. That includes your rent, your business rates, your water, your electricity, your computer system and so on. That's everything that you need to spend for your business to function. Those are your basic breakeven costs.

Once you've worked those out, look at wages and the cost of your staff. You need to know how much each person needs to bring in to not only cover their wages, but also to cover the cost of having them there providing services at your salon as well as added profits.

One of the tools our Salon Jedis love is our hourly rate calculator. Once you add your expenses, it totals your breakeven figure. You then add your number of stylists and/or therapists (even if it's just you), the hours available, and then the profit percentage you want to make, and it calculates the hourly rate you should be charging. It's a great tool for when your breakeven, team levels and utilisation fluctuates so you can keep an eye on your hourly rate to make sure you're still on track and profitable. If this sounds like something you'd find useful, use the contact details at the end of the book to arrange a call with us.

YOU GET MORE OF WHAT YOU FOCUS ON

As I've said already in this book, you get more of what you focus on. In my experience, the more you track your targets, the more you're able to hit them. One of my top tips is to break your targets down into manageable amounts. Work out your annual sales target, for example, but then break this down into weekly amounts to make it manageable.

It's also important that you recognise that tracking negative outcomes can lead to those expanding. For example, at one point I noticed that our team were taking quite a lot of sick days, so I started tracking staff absences. All that happened was that people started taking more sick days. This comes back to mindset, so I switched my thinking and started tracking the reduction in sick days across the team, and sure enough the number of people taking time off due to illness fell.

It's the same when you're tracking wastage. You want to track the reduction in stock wastage, rather than the amount that is being wasted. Tracking and measuring your numbers is just one side of it, because you have to make sure that you're focusing on tracking the right metrics and that you're tracking them in the direction that you want them to be going in.

For example, when we track the wastage from hair colours, all the dye that's left over goes into a tub and that gets weighed each day. We then calculate the cost per weight of that product so we can get a reasonably accurate idea of how much stock is being wasted. You might discover that you're wasting £50 per week and when you multiply that up over a year, it equates to £2,600.

When you've got those figures you can go back to your team and explain why it's important to focus on reducing waste and you can find a way to do that. You can also incentivise them to focus on reducing waste. For example, you might say that if they save that £2,600 you're going to use a percentage of that money to pay for a trip to a training event. Again, this comes back to mindset. You're not just telling them to avoid wastage to make more money for the business, you're showing them what's in it for them (the WIIFM rule).

This is all about tracking your numbers in the right way. As I've said many times, you get more of what you focus on. If you're reading this book and you know that every week your target is to break even, I can tell you now that you're only breaking even each week and you won't do anything other than break even unless you change your focus.

USE YOUR NUMBERS TO IDENTIFY THE HOLES IN YOUR BUCKET

I'm sure you've heard of the leaky bucket concept, where you're pouring water into the top but it's leaking out of the holes at the bottom. When you start to really focus on and understand your numbers you will start to identify the holes in your bucket. This will allow you to work out where you need to put your focus in order to plug those holes and help you retain more water in your bucket.

There is no single way to approach your figures because every salon is different and you need to look at all of the variables that affect your business. If this is an area you know you're struggling with, it's important that you get some support to start exploring how to better track and measure the figures that are important in your business.

It's never going to hurt to get someone from outside your business to go through your figures with you.

If you are still in doubt about the importance of getting to grips with your numbers, look at me as an example. Numbers aren't my strength, but when I started focusing on them and finding simple formulas and simple ways of working that worked for me, I saw a huge difference in my business. My business consistently makes a good profit, year in, year out. We've got some stylists who have taken up to £6,500 in one week and we have a 99% attendance rate for our staff. Those are the kinds of figures you can achieve when you not only focus on your numbers, but when you focus on those numbers moving in the right direction.

EXERCISE

For me, the key to getting to grips with my numbers has been to simplify everything as much as possible. If you've read this chapter and feel like you don't know where to start, I would recommend a simple formula as a target, but remember that all salons are different. You can start by setting your target for your takings at 2.5 times your wage bill as an estimate.

That's not set in stone, but it will give you a starting point if this is a completely new area to you. For an example of our figures model and pie model, scan the QR code below.

CHAPTER 15

SCALE TO EXIT

As you're coming to the end of the book, we've covered the four areas that you need to master to be able to scale your salon business: mindset, marketing, management and maintenance. Mastering all of these will also put you in a strong position should you wish to exit, but you might not want to. For you, scaling your business might be the most important thing. Or you might just want to have one really solid, profitable salon that allows you to take a step back and enjoy your life. Whatever end goal you have in mind, following these steps will allow you to create a salon business that is not dependent on you as the operator.

This is a really key point to remember: when you are an owner not an operator, your business is more profitable and therefore it's more valuable should you wish to sell it.

I started at the beginning of the book with the example of the two salon owners to show you how important having the right mindset is. My own story and the success of my salon is living proof of that as well. You have to remember that your salon is a reflection of you, and your mindset is the foundation of everything that follows. If you have all the other pieces but not that one, you're much less likely to achieve the success you're aiming for.

Marketing is all about your clients and attracting the right clients to your business. When you get this right, you will bring in more of your ideal clients, but to do that you have to get your foundation in place because this is what attracts them to your salon.

Management focuses on the customer care journey and making sure that your team are doing everything you need them to do to delight your clients and drive the business forward. This all comes from the culture you've created in your salon and is a reflection of you and your core values. As a salon owner, there are many variables that you have to manage and getting the management right is essential if you're going to provide the level of care you need to keep your customers coming back.

Finally, we've talked about maintenance and the importance of maintaining everything you've put in place. You can do an excellent job on those first three stages, but if you fail to maintain everything you've set up, you'll see standards and service start to slide. Gradually that will chip away at the profitability of the business you've worked so hard to build.

Those are the four key building blocks to creating a sustainable, sound, profitable business that you're able to scale and eventually exit if you want to. With these building blocks in place, you can give yourself more freedom and you have a choice of where you go next.

WHY CONSIDER SCALING TO EXIT?

You might be reading this and thinking that you don't want to exit your business and you can't imagine ever reaching the point where you will want to. That's fine. I'm not saying that this is a step that you have to take, but implementing everything I've talked about up to this point will give you the choice.

Do you remember the part of my story that I shared right at the beginning of this book, where I was crying in my staffroom because I'd just been told my business was worth nothing and I felt trapped? Scaling your business, systemising it and giving yourself greater freedom from the salon means you'll never be in that position. You will always have the choice of selling your business, because you've made it profitable and sustainable without you being there.

MY STORY

WHY I SACKED MYSELF FROM THE SALON FLOOR

Even though I don't work on the salon floor any longer, unless it's a VIP client, I'm still hugely passionate about the industry. I love the creative side of hairdressing and this is an area that I'm still involved in at the salon and I still love this role as Creative Director. I've been on a wonderful journey in this industry, but sacking myself from the salon floor the majority of the time was what I needed to do to follow my new passion. I wanted to give my team the chance to rise up and grow. I wanted to see them being excited about following their own career paths, having full columns and being promoted. I wanted to see my budding salon manager flourish and have the freedom to grow. I find my joy and passion now in helping others develop the business side of their salons. Fundamentally what my mindset, marketing, management and maintenance have given me is the freedom to follow my own purpose. That's what I want to help you do, whatever your purpose may be.

MULTIPLY YOUR IMPACT ON THE WORLD

If you're able to build a business that works, as much as possible, without you, then you have this incredible freedom to step away. You don't have a job any more, you're not trading your time for money, instead you're able to build that profitable business and then use your time to multiply your impact on the world. Just think of how many more people you could help if you were able to take a step back from your business and have a bit more time.

What impact you choose to have is entirely up to you. The point is you're able to help other people; and even just by having a profitable and stable business you're helping people because you're giving people jobs, you're training people and helping them progress to become managers, and you're putting a culture in place at your salon that has a positive impact on your customers. It's all about this ripple effect and, for me, it's wonderful to know that I'm having that impact without having to be in my business every day.

FOCUS ON HELPING, NOT ON CONTROLLING

If you're building a business that will give you more freedom to pursue your passions, you have to let go of control. Focus on helping everyone on your team to perform at their best and to build amazing careers, but let go of the control. This is about putting all the tools and systems that I've talked about in place so that your salon, or salons, can run smoothly without you.

If you don't have the foundations that I've talked about in this book firmly in place, you'll just find that you're constantly drawn back into the business to deal with problems.

REVISIT YOUR VISION

When you reach the stage where you're thinking about scaling, or starting to scale, your business, or where you're exploring the possibility of exiting your business, come back to your vision. Does the vision you set out at the beginning align with where you are now? Everyone has their own mission or vision and for some of you that might be to have one profitable lifestyle salon, but I would challenge you to think bigger.

As I discussed in the mindset part of the book, a lot of the time we set targets based on what we think we can achieve, and that can limit us. When you're working really hard to build one successful salon, it can be very easy to focus on the stress and the problems you might be experiencing and think that if you scale, that will only introduce more problems; but that's only going to be true if you're the only one who's doing everything.

Many of the salon owners I work with at the start are doing so much that they feel torn between the different elements of their business, or between their salons if they have more than one. This is why getting the right team in place is so important if you want to scale. You need to get the right people in the right seats doing the right job – you don't have to do everything yourself. You need to know that you've put the right systems in place and that you've hired the right person for the job, and then you'll be able to release control.

ADDING VALUE TO YOUR SALON

Every salon owner wants to have a profitable business and even if you're not thinking about exiting your business now, at some stage you are likely to reach a point where you want to exit, even if that's just to fully retire.

What you're doing by putting the foundations of mindset, marketing, management and maintenance in place is adding value to your salon. Implementing systems, hiring a high-performing team, creating a culture and a brand that appeals to customers, having a predictable income, automating your marketing: all of these elements add value to a business to someone looking at it from the outside. This comes back to the concept that you want to be an owner not an operator. Will the business still run smoothly and profitably without you? If you've done everything I've talked about in this book then the answer is yes. Even if that's not what you want for your business right now, it's about knowing you have the option if you want to take it.

Statistics show only 10% of businesses registered for sale will sell. Don't be a statistic where you end up in a position where you NEED to sell, like I was back in 2009.

I'm living proof that everything I've talked about in this book works. You've read my story and you know that I have turned my salon around from a 'worthless' business to one that's now turning over hundreds of thousands of pounds a year. The reason I focus on mindset, marketing, management and maintenance is because they work, and the reason I know they work is because I've used them to build my business.

The results from 2019 speak for themselves, and please note as you read them that they were achieved with only four to five stylists and me off the tools:

- Highest turnover for our salon and academy: £627,904.49
- Highest ever 6 figure profits
- Highest salon takings in one month: £52,809.78
- Highest salon takings in one week: £24,236.39
- Highest-performing stylist: £6,650 (one week)/£15,019 (one month)
- Highest Facebook reach: 1,107,849 people
- Highest views on one video: 156,060
- Staff attendance rate: 99% (zero sick days for most)
- Care factor: 22% (percentage of clients who leave with retail)
- Retail income: up 28%
- Retail units sold: up 23.5%
- New salon clients: 1,345
- Salon Elite Memberships: 22% (up 120%)
- Marketing spend: 1,047% ROI (return on investment)

> 'Caroline and her team have bagged over 100 award nominations and wins and 2020 sees the launch of her *M.I.N.D.F.U.L.* Salon Source Code, teaching salons a 4-part solution covering mindset, marketing, management and maintenance to grow their business and put systems in place to ensure ongoing success without salon owners having to be on the salon floor to oversee everything.'
>
> \- **Salonnv.co.uk**

MULTIPLYING MY IMPACT: SALON JEDI ACADEMY

My passion for multiplying my impact is what led me to create the Salon Jedi Academy. Realising the power of the knowledge I'd built up from building my business was what inspired me to establish our Salon Jedi Academy ten years ago. I realised that there were many other salon owners who had been in a similar position to me and who would benefit from guidance and support to develop and grow their businesses.

Through Salon Jedi, I've been able to help owners master their mindsets to take control of their salons, build high-performing teams and create highly profitable businesses that allow them to release themselves from the tools more and follow their purpose; be it expanding the business, creating an academy or something outside of the industry.

At the Academy we offer different levels of training, which allows you to work at your own pace. We offer individual digital training courses, live and digital events, live three-day courses, where we run through much of what's in this book in more detail, as well as two-day salon transformations for those in the UK, where we visit your salon and look at your business on a deeper level and help you plug in our systems. We run year-long digital academy programmes with coaching, as well as our LITE Academy low monthly membership. Whatever form of training you choose to follow, you have to have space to learn. It takes time to get your mindset in place and lay that foundation, but once you start implementing and getting things right you can look to accelerate and then leverage what you're doing at your business.

You've heard about some of the results salon owners have seen from joining my training programmes as you've read this book. With some help and guidance, you can build your salon into the business you've always wanted it to be and find the freedom to follow your passions.

I have worked with the best mindset mentors across the globe, including a year-long mastermind with John Assaraf, courses with Dr Demartini, one-to-one coaching with Andy Harrington (who wrote the foreword for the book); and have trained in person with some of the best marketers on the planet, including Chris Cardel, Dan Kennedy and Einstein Marketer Mat Wilson. I bring this knowledge back to my own salon and test and implement it before sharing it with my students across the globe.

I don't just teach theory, I am teaching what I do so others can follow and learn proven strategies.

If you'd like to learn more about the programmes, training and coaching I offer through my Salon Jedi Academy, get in touch: info@salonjedimarketing.com

As you can see from reading this book, the strategies that we use at Salon Jedi work amazingly well. You just need to look at the testimonials at the front of this book and the case studies from Chris and Emma, Krysia, and Lisa, as well as my own results, to see that the strategies work.

- In just six years, Chris and Emma went from being over £10,000 overdrawn to having a positive balance of around £90,000 in their business account.
- Krysia made £25,000 in just one day using one of Caroline's marketing strategies.
- In only six months with the Salon Jedi Academy, Lisa has been able to come off the tools to work ON her business rather than IN it.
- At Ego Hair Design, our marketing spend delivers at 1,047% ROI and we attracted 1,345 new salon clients with our unique marketing strategies.

As a reward for reading this book, I would like to invite you to book a free one-hour breakthrough discovery call. This breakthrough call is to look inside your business to see how to improve profits, scalability and leverage, and to identify any limiting beliefs holding you back.

We will help you discover what is not working in your salon business and plan how to scale up and reach your dream profits, even while getting off the tools if you wish.

This is a part of our mission at Salon Jedi to reach and teach 7,500 salon professionals across the globe to help them grow their business and make a positive impact on the world in their own way.

To book, simply scan the QR code below with your mobile phone's camera and choose a time that works for you.

If you keep doing what you've always done, you will keep getting the same results. While I know first-hand it can be daunting, in the words of Martin Luther King Jr, 'You don't have to see the whole staircase, just take the first step.'

Find us on social media
Facebook: @salonjedi @carsanderson
Instagram: @thesalonjedi @sanderson_caroline
Tiktok: SalonJedi
LinkedIn: /Carolinesanderson1

ABOUT THE AUTHOR

Caroline is Salon Director of Ego Hair Design in Inverness, Scotland, and Director of the Salon Jedi Academy, an international salon business training academy for salon owners who want to improve their businesses. The digital Salon Jedi Academy is also the first (and at the time of writing only) digital training academy to be awarded a five star Good Training Guide accreditation from the Good Salon Guide.

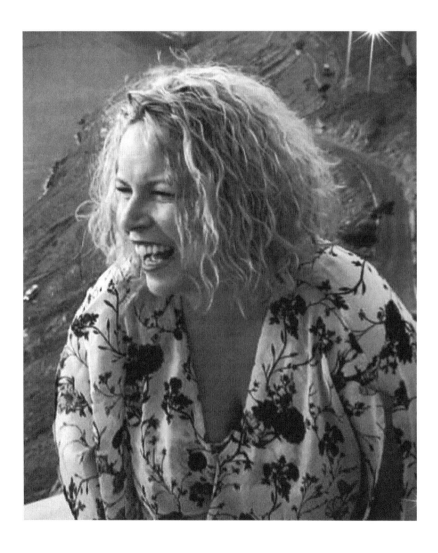

Caroline, her team and her businesses have won over 100 awards and nominations, including Creative HEAD's Most Wanted Awards, British Hairdressing Awards and British Hairdressing Business Awards, as well as being nominated for Great British Creative Entrepreneur of the Year.

Caroline's purpose is to empower ambitious salon owners to become masters of their minds and businesses for more profits and freedom. She has a burning belief that people are more capable than they give themselves credit for and, having struggled with her own salon herself, Caroline is perfectly placed to help other salon owners unlock their potential. She strongly believes that if she can do this, then anyone can, as long as they have the right guidance.

When she's not teaching or creating, Caroline loves spending time with her children. She also spends a lot of time reading, listening to audiobooks and meditating – what she describes as 'growing the brain'.

Caroline lives in Inverness with her three children. They're her big 'Why' and her desire to build a secure future for them is what set her off on the journey towards creating and building Ego Hair Design and the Salon Jedi Academy.

Accreditations:

Member of the Fellowship of British Hairdressing
The first 5 Star Good Training Guide Accreditation for a digital academy
Certified to practice NLP and Ho'oponopono
Graduate of Public Speakers University
BHA Hons in Fine Art
Currently studying Diplomas in Jungian Archetypes, Mastering Flow State, Mindfulness and Mindful Mental Health

Printed in Great Britain
by Amazon